About the publisher

BPP Learning Media is dedicated to supporting aspiring professionals with top quality learning material. BPP Learning Media's commitment to success is shown by our record of quality, innovation and market leadership in paper-based and e-learning materials. BPP Learning Media's study materials are written by professionally-qualified specialists who know from personal experience the importance of top quality materials for success.

About The BMJ

The BMJ (formerly the British Medical Journal) in print has a long history and has been published without interruption since 1840. The BMJ's vision is to be the world's most influential and widely read medical journal. Our mission is to lead the debate on health and to engage, inform, and stimulate doctors, researchers, and other health professionals in ways that will improve outcomes for patients. We aim to help doctors to make better decisions. BMJ, the company, advances healthcare worldwide by sharing knowledge and expertise to improve experiences, outcomes and value.

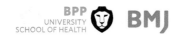

Contents

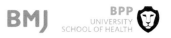

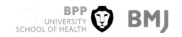

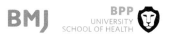

About the editors

Professor Adrian Hunnisett is a biomedical scientist specialising in clinical biochemistry and haematology. He completed initial BMS training at Gloucester Royal Hospital and then graduated from Oxford Brookes University, completing research training in Oxford and London. He has worked in a variety of roles within the NHS and private medical sectors, most recently as Head of Clinical R&D at Southampton General Hospital. He is now Professor of Evidence-Based Healthcare at BPP University.

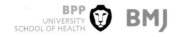

Introduction to Research Methods and Reporting series

As a healthcare worker, you are working in an "evidence-based" or "evidence-informed" professional environment whatever your professional discipline, whether you are doctors, nurses, physiotherapists, occupational therapist or part of the emerging plethora of allied professions. The evidence you use, the research base, is being generated constantly and that is impacting on clinical practice at all levels. The information you all learned in your clinical training has rapidly, and inevitably, become outdated. As a result there is a clear need to understand the principles of research and research methods to help you make decisions about the mass of new knowledge and integrating it into your practice whilst discontinuing the "old traditions".

Over recent years, the teaching of clinical research methods, research practice and the evaluation of clinical evidence has become a core addition to undergraduate and postgraduate curricula across all healthcare disciplines. In addition, many clinical journals have articles and sections concentrating on continuing education providing tools for reading and critiquing the vast amount of emerging research. Such material is considered so important in the development of evidence-based practice that they may attract credits toward the CPD portfolios required by many of the professional registration bodies today.

The BMJ Research Methods & Reporting books bring together a collection of review articles first published in the British Medical Journal. They are not designed to replace the basic knowledge of research methods and evaluation, but rather to answer some of the key questions that researchers at all levels ask along with updates in the reporting structures and regulations for articles in the medical press. Each of the articles is written by acknowledged experts in their fields and they offer a broad update on many aspects of research, research methodology and guidelines for undertaking and reporting research. They are written in a user-friendly way that is easy to follow and understand by the non-specialist. In addition, each article is fully referenced with links to further information and evidence to support the statements made in the article. The collections are aimed at non-specialist doctors, general practitioners, research nurses and healthcare practitioners. They can also be used by individuals who may be preparing for any postgraduate examinations that have a research element.

There are two separate volumes, each concentrating on a different aspect of the research process. The first volume examines some key messages about the basics of research along with up to date articles on statistical approaches, methods and interpretation. The topics covered concentrate on subjects such as confidence intervals, p values, sample size calculations, use of patient reported outcome measures, conundrums in the application of RCT and more complex statistical analysis. It also highlights implementation research and prognostic research. The second is more specific with articles on the reporting requirements for research. It examines guidelines such as CONSORT, SPIRIT, GPP2, PRISMA and the IDEAL framework for surgical innovation. It also gives some guidance on economic evaluations, policy and service interventions and publication guidelines, as well as providing useful tips on preparing data for publication.

Each book is a stand-alone volume, but together they will give the reader a comprehensive overview of the commoner research issues and guidelines.

Adrian Hunnisett (November 2015).

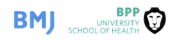

Sample size calculations: should the emperor's clothes be off the peg or made to measure?

Geoffrey Norman, statistician and cognitive psychologist[1],
Sandra Monteiro, graduate student[2],
Suzette Salama, chair of McMaster research ethics board[3]

...ical Epidemiology and ...tatistics, McMaster University, ...L 3519, 1280 Main St W, ...ilton, Ontario L8S 2T1, Canada

...artment of Psychology, ...aster University, Hamilton

...dicine, Hamilton Health ...nces, Hamilton

...espondence to: G Norman
...man@mcmaster.ca

this as: BMJ 2012;345:e5278

10.1136/bmj.e5278

...//www.bmj.com/content/345/
e5278

Conventional wisdom dictates that it is unethical to conduct a study that is so large that excess numbers of patients are exposed or so small that clinically important changes cannot be detected.[1] This implies that there is some optimal sample size that can be calculated using statistical theory and information from previous research. But the choice of sample size is usually a compromise between statistical considerations, which always benefit from increased sample size, and economic or logistical constraints.[2]

Only rarely is sufficient information available to make informed decisions. Moreover, despite the illusion of precision that arises from the application of arcane statistical formulas, in many situations the choice of inputs—the expected treatment effect, the standard deviation, and the power—are subject to considerable uncertainty. As a result, sample size calculations may vary widely.

We argue that, in the absence of good data, it would be better to determine sample size by adopting norms derived from historical data based on large numbers of studies of the same type. We show that for many common situations we can define defensible, evidence based, ranges of sample sizes.

An example
Imagine that you decide to do a study to see if control of primary hypertension is improved by home monitoring. You visit your local statistician for a sample size calculation, as the ethics board insists. The following are some key questions that he or she will ask and some tentative answers.

What is the distribution of blood pressure in the population you intend to study?
One study design might be to randomise people to treatment and control groups, put one group on monitors for a few months, then measure their blood pressure. We would then compare blood pressure in the two groups. To compute sample size, we need to know the standard deviation of systolic (or diastolic) blood pressure in the group we are studying. One recent meta-analysis of interventions to control hypertension gave values of 15-17 mm Hg.[3]

ABSTRACT

Ethics committees require estimates of sample size for all trials, but statistical calculations are no more accurate than estimates from historical data. **Geoffrey Norman and colleagues** propose some "one size fits all" numbers for different study designs

How much do you think your treatment will affect systolic blood pressure?
The most reasonable answer is, "How do I know? That's why I'm doing the study." Regrettably, you have to know to calculate sample size. Fortunately, a recent Cochrane review of 12 randomised trials with over 1200 patients per group provides a guide.[3] The mean difference in systolic pressure was 2.53 mm Hg. Individual study results ranged from a drop of 26.0 mm Hg to a gain of 5.0 mm Hg. If we eliminate the two studies with very small samples of 9 and 18 and use the three largest observed differences, we end up with a mean drop of 6.9 mm Hg from studies with samples of 48, 55, and 76. Conversely, the studies with the three smallest treatment effects (n=123, 326, and 72) showed an average benefit of 1 mm Hg.

What α and β levels do you want?
That's easy. Convention dictates that α (level of statistical significance) is 0.05 and β (the probability of a type II error: accepting the null hypothesis when the alternate hypothesis is true) is 0.20. (However easy and universal these may be, the choice of a power of 0.80 is logically unsupportable, as shown by Bacchetti.[2] But for the sake of convention, we will proceed.)

We can now do the calculation (box). If we take the extremes, the smallest sample size, based on a reduction of 6.9 mm Hg and an SD of 15, equals 75 per group. The largest, for a 1 mm Hg drop and an SD of 17, equals 4624. The overall average drop of 2.53 corresponds to a sample size of 722. These estimates differ by a factor of 60 even though this was a "best case" situation, in which all studies had reasonable sample size and were viewed as sufficiently homogeneous to be included in a systematic review.

Critics might argue that the choice of the three smallest and largest differences was arbitrary and extreme, but we used it to illustrate the point. We could have used alternative strategies, such as weighting by sample size. But the fact is that all the studies were derived from a Cochrane systematic review, all were examining a single question, all were deemed of sufficient quality to be included in the systematic review, and all were used in the final calculation in the review. On that basis, all are equal candidates for inclusion in a sample size calculation.

SUMMARY POINTS

Conventional sample size calculations, based on guesses about statistical parameters, are subject to large uncertainties

There is sufficient evidence to justify establishing expected normative ranges of sample sizes for common research designs

Normative ranges can be modified if good evidence exists on which to base a sample size calculation

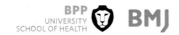

In more representative situations where data are lacking, there would be even more "wiggle room." Virtually all statisticians who have been engaged in this activity describe multiple iterations until the computed sample size converges to a desired result.

Other approaches to sample size

Interestingly, inclusion of sample size as an element of research ethics is far more pervasive in health sciences than in other areas such as social sciences. In Canada, the authoritative Tricouncil statement on ethics—produced by the three federal research councils for health, social sciences, and physical science—mentions sample size only in the section on qualitative research. In non-medical disciplines it seems that judgments about adequacy of sample size, if raised at all, are resolved by arguments along the lines of "studies in this area typically use sample sizes about this large." Perhaps this is because biomedical research is more likely to expose participants to real, occasionally life threatening, risks.

Clinical trials also typically include large numbers of people, and the cost per person is high. All these factors increase pressure to arrive at the "right" sample size. However, as Bacchetti argues, any sample size is a compromise and high risks and costs really should be seen as factors to reduce sample size.[2]

Calculation of sample size seems unlikely to disappear, whatever the philosophical flaws in the argument. But in view of the imprecision of the estimates, we need a fundamental rethink of the approach to avoid the calculation being seen (with justification) as simply another hoop to jump through to obtain ethical approval.

We propose a new approach that establishes norms for particular study questions and designs, while not preventing the investigator from producing an individual estimate when the evidence warrants it. The idea stems from a proposal by Bacchetti[2] and from the commonsense idea to use existing data when available to increase precision of estimates.

As we have seen, individual estimates, even when based on previous studies, can vary wildly. Still, it is a large leap of faith to presume that "cultural" norms based on previous research are more defensible. However, in some areas there is good evidence of the magnitude of treatment effects that might be expected. For studies of two groups in which the outcome is either a measured (interval or ratio) dependent variable or a difference in proportions, we argue that there is sufficient evidence from various sources to compute norms for sample sizes that may apply to all such studies. For some regression methods, there are "rules of thumb" that do not require specific information.

Sample size norms for different designs

Differences between groups

Measured outcome variable
The most basic study design on which to base a sample size calculation resembles our introductory example. Participants are assigned to two groups: one group receives a treatment and the other a placebo, the outcome is measured on a continuous scale (such as blood pressure, range of motion, creatinine concentration), and the means of the two groups are compared.

> **CALCULATING SAMPLE SIZE**
>
> For a difference between two groups, sample size=$16 \times s^2/d^2$ where s is the standard deviation and d is the expected treatment effect.
>
> As Lehr has shown,[4] for α=0.05 and power of 0.80 this is a close approximation to the exact formula. We have deliberate[ly] rounded the computed values to avoid the illusion of precision.

The classic text for sample size and power calculati[on] is Cohen's *Statistical Power Analysis for the Behavio[ral] Sciences*.[5] The basis for the sample size calculation is [the] effect size—the treatment difference divided by the standa[rd] deviation within groups. Based on his experience, Co[hen] proposed that a small effect size is 0.2, a medium is [0.5] and a large is 0.8. On this basis, the norm for sample si[ze] would be 400, 64, and 25 respectively.

Although equating of 0.2, 0.5, and 0.8 with small, medi[um,] and large effect sizes has now become almost axiomatic, Co[hen] did not view them that way.[2] He spends considerable t[ime] arguing the reasonableness of these estimates by compar[ing] them with other indices such as overlap of distributio[ns,] correlations, and percent of variance, as well as ancho[ring] to commonly accepted scales like intelligence quotient ([IQ.] Halpern went further and argued that, in the absence of [any] more specific data, sample size could be based on a medi[um] effect size (0.5), so the default would be n=64.[6]

We are not suggesting that sample size estimates sho[uld] be based on small, medium, or large effect sizes. Rather [we] should use norms within research communities—explic[itly] using archival data to identify representative and expec[ted] normative values of effect size. As one example, Lipsey a[nd] Wilson examined 302 meta-analyses of 13 000 studies look[ing] at educational and psychological interventions.[7] They fou[nd] a mean effect across all studies of 0.50, with a standa[rd] deviation of 0.29. This large series is quite consistent w[ith] Cohen's original estimates and results in a sample s[ize] between 26 and 363, again with a best estimate of 64.

Another approach to sample size calculation involv[es] consideration of the minimally important difference (M[ID).] There are several approaches to determining the MID, m[ost] commonly by observing change in a cohort of patients w[ho] are judged to have had minimal change in their qua[lity] of life. One study looked at 38 studies estimating the M[ID] in health related quality of life.[8] The mean MID over [all] estimates was 0.495, with an SD of 0.15. From this surv[ey] the range of sample sizes (±1SD) would be 38 to 134, w[ith] a best estimate of 65.

Both these examples estimate that a study with t[wo] groups and a continuous outcome might use a sample s[ize] of about 60 per group, although anything within the ran[ge] 25 to 400 is acceptable, with larger samples for treatme[nt-] treatment comparisons and smaller samples for comparis[ons] with no treatment. They also happen to be consistent w[ith] Cohen's medium effect size, although this cannot be se[en] as justification to adopt 0.5 as a standard since ma[ny] clinical interventions have much smaller effect sizes.[7]

Binary outcome variable— proportions
Many clinical trials use a binary (death/no death, eve[nt/] no event) outcome. The sample size formula differs and [is] dependent on both the base rate of the outcome and t[he] risk reduction. If we can establish a normative range [of] relative risk reduction to be expected, then a sample s[ize] curve, describing the sample size for a particular base ra[te] can be easily produced.

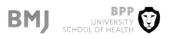

Table | Sample sizes for various combinations of relative risk reduction and base rate*

Base rate	Relative risk reduction		
	0.08	0.16	0.25
0.01	247 500	61875	25300
0.02	122500	30625	12550
0.05	47500	11875	4 865
0.1	22500	5625	2 300
0.2	10000	2 500	1025
0.5	2 500	625	255

*Sample size based on the approximate formula $n=16\times(BR(1-BR))/ARR^2$, where BR=base rate and ARR=absolute risk reduction. Sample sizes are rounded to the nearest 5 or 0.

Is it plausible that most trials will have risk reductions within a narrow range? Yusuf has argued this case and has produced evidence from 42 cardiovascular trials of chronic interventions (such as aspirin) and 84 trials of acute interventions (such as intravenous nitrates).[9] Relative risk reductions ranged from 8% to 36% (mean 15%) for the chronic interventions and 6% to 24% (mean 19%) for the acute interventions. Averaging all studies, the mean relative risk reduction was 16.5% (SD 8.4%). The table shows sample sizes for base rates of 2%, 5%, 10%, and 20% using an adapted sample size formula. Though the variation in sample size overall is very large, from 250 to 19 800 per group, for a particular base rate, the range of sample sizes reduces to roughly 10 to one.

Relations between continuous variables

The relation between two continuous variables can be assessed with the correlation coefficient. The standard error of the correlation is roughly $(1-r^2)/(n-2)$. If we assume that typical correlations are in the range of 0.2 to 0.5, then with $\alpha=0.05$ and a power of 0.80 the estimated sample size $(n=2+8\times(1-r^2)/r^2)$ ranges from 44 to 194. Why 0.2 to 0.5? Pragmatism. A correlation of less than 0.2 accounts for less than 4% of the variance; a correlation of 0.1 accounts for only 1%. It is difficult to imagine why anyone would care about a relation that explains less than 4%. On the other hand, correlations greater than 0.5 are fairly rare and researchers would be unlikely to design a study in the hope of detecting a correlation this large. With these bounds, we might accept any sample size in the range 50-200.

For multivariable analyses such as multiple regression, logistic regression, and factor analysis, everything depends on everything else. No exact predictions are really feasible. Consequently, rules of thumb are often adopted that the sample size should be 5, 10, or 20 times the number of variables. The maths is therefore simple: for five predictors, sample sizes of 25 might be acceptable, and a sample size of 100 would meet the most stringent rule of thumb.

Conclusions

Sample size estimates are like the emperor's clothes; we collectively act in public as if they possess an impressive aura of precision, yet privately we (statisticians) are acutely aware of their shortcomings and extreme imprecision. Clearly, all would benefit from a new approach. In many circumstances, researchers should be encouraged to use the "off the peg" sample sizes we have suggested, although a "made to measure" calculation can be used if sufficient information is available to justify it. More generally, we support the position of Bacchetti[2] that any attempt to determine a precise sample size must necessarily consider more than simple numerical issues and should explicitly deal with broader ethical issues underlying the choice.

Competing interests: All authors have completed the ICMJE unified disclosure form at www.icmje.org/coi_disclosure.pdf (available on request from the corresponding author) and declare GN is funded by a Canada research chair; they have no financial relationships with any organisations that might have an interest in the submitted work in the previous three years and no other relationships or activities that could appear to have influenced the submitted work.

Contributors: GN did the calculations and was primarily responsible for writing the paper. SS suggested the topic and reviewed and critiqued multiple drafts. SM conducted literature searches, and reviewed and contributed to drafts of the paper. GN is guarantor.

Provenance and peer review: Not commissioned; externally peer reviewed.

1   Altman DG. Why we need confidence intervals. *World J Surg* 2005;29:554-6.
2   Bacchetti P. Current sample size conventions: flaws, harms, and alternatives. *BMC Med* 2010;8:17.
3   Glynn LG, Murphy AW, Smith SM, Schroeder K, Fahey T. Interventions used to improve control of blood pressure in patients with hypertension. *Cochrane Database Syst Rev* 2010;3:CD005182.
4   Lehr R. Sixteen S-squared over D-squared: a relation for crude sample size estimates. *Stat Med* 1992;11:1099-102.
5   Cohen JJ. Statistical power analysis for the behavioral sciences. Erlbaum, 1988.
6   Halpern SD, Karlawish JHT, Berlin JA. The continuing unethical conduct of underpowered clinical trials. *JAMA* 2002;288:358-62.
7   Lipsey MW, Wilson DB. The efficacy of psychological, educational, and behavioral treatment. Confirmation from meta-analysis. *Am Psychol* 1993;48:1181-209.
8   Norman GR, Sloan JA, Wyrwich KW. Interpretation of changes in health-related quality of life: the remarkable universality of half a standard deviation. *Med Care* 2003;41:582-92.
9   Yusuf S, Collins R, Peto R. Why do we need some large, simple randomized trials? *Stat Med* 1984;3:409-22.

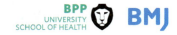

The tyranny of power: is there a better way to calculate sample size?

John Martin Bland, professor of health statistics

Department of Health Sciences, University of York, Heslington, York YO10 5DD

mb55@york.ac.uk

Cite this as: *BMJ* 2009;339:b3985

DOI: 10.1136/bmj.b3985

http://www.bmj.com/content/339/bmj.b3985

When I began my career in medical statistics, back in 1972, little was heard of power calculations. In major journals, sample size often seemed to be whatever came to hand. For example, in September 1972, the *Lancet* contained 31 research reports that used individual subject data, excluding case reports and animal studies. The median sample size was 33 (quartiles 12 and 85). In the same month the *BMJ* had 30 reports of the same type, with median sample size 37 (quartiles 12 and 158). None of these publications explained the choice of sample size, other than it being what was available. Indeed, statistical considerations were almost entirely lacking from the methods sections of these papers.

Compare the research papers of September 1972 with those in the same journals in September 2007, 35 years later. In the *Lancet*, there were 14 such research reports, with median sample size 3116 (quartiles 1246 and 5584), two orders of magnitude greater than in 1972. In September 2007, the *BMJ* carried 12 such research reports, with median sample size 3104 (quartiles 236 and 23351). Power calculations were reported for four of the *Lancet* papers and five of the *BMJ* papers.

The patterns in the two journals are strikingly similar. For each journal, sample sizes increased almost a 100-fold, the proportion of papers reporting power calculations increased from none to one third, and the number of studies of individual participants was less than half that in 1972. The difference in the number of reports is not because of the number of issues; in both years, September was a five issue month. I suggest that the changes in sample size result from the adoption of power calculations.

Power calculations

In the past there were problems arising from what now seem to be very small sample sizes. Studies were typically analysed using significance tests, and differences were often not significant. What does "not significant" mean? It means that we have not found evidence against the null hypothesis—for example, that there is no evidence for a difference between two types of treatments. This was often misinterpreted as meaning that there was no difference. Potentially valuable treatments were being rejected and potentially harmful ones were not being replaced. I recall Richard Peto presenting a (never published) study of expert opinion on three approaches to the treatment of myocardial infarction, as expressed in leading articles in

ABSTRACT

Martin Bland's extensive experience in reviewing and using power calculations has led him to believe that it is time to replace them

the *New England Journal of Medicine* and the *Lancet*, and contrasting this with the exactly opposite conclusions that he had drawn from a systematic review and meta-analysis of all published randomised trials in these areas.

Acknowledgment of the problems with small samples led to changes. One of these was the advance calculation of sample size to try to ensure that a study would answer its question. The method that has been almost universally adopted reflects the significance level approach to analysis, the so called power calculation. (In practice, power is seldom calculated, though it is used. It is chosen by the researchers in advance, usually to be 0.90 or 0.80.)

The idea of statistical power is deceptively simple. We are going to do a study where we will evaluate the evidence using a significance test. We decide what the outcome variable is going to be and what the comparison is going to be. For example, the outcome variable might be systolic blood pressure and the comparison would be between mean blood pressure in two groups. We then decide what the test of significance would be, such as a two sample *t* test comparing mean systolic pressure. We decide how big a difference we want the study to detect—that is, how big a difference would be worth knowing about. For a two sample *t* test of mean systolic pressure, this could be the difference in mean pressure that would lead us to adopt the new treatment. We then choose a sample size so that if this difference were the actual difference in the population, a large proportion of possible samples would produce a statistically significant difference. This proportion is the power.

Statistical formulas to determine power for different significance tests are incorporated in many computer programs, both specialist sample size software and some general statistical packages. For many of these calculations we need to supply some other information about the outcome variable. For mean blood pressure, we would also require the standard deviation of blood pressure measurements in the population we wish to study. To compare two proportions, we would need to supply the expected proportion in one of the groups in addition to the difference between them.

There are problems with power calculations, however, even for simple studies. To do them, we require some knowledge of the research area. For example, if we wish to compare two means, we need an idea of the variability of the quantity being measured, such as its standard deviation; if we wish to compare two proportions, we need an estimate of the proportion in the control group. We might reasonably expect researchers to have this knowledge, but it is surprising how often they do not. We are then reduced to saying that we could hope to detect a difference of

SUMMARY POINTS

- Most medical research studies have sample sizes justified by power calculations
- Power calculations are based on significance tests
- Many journals require results to be presented with confidence intervals
- Sample size calculations should be based on the width of a confidence interval, not power

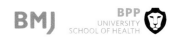

some specified fraction of a standard deviation. Cohen[1] has dignified this by the name "effect size," but the name is often a cloak for ignorance.

If we know enough about our research area to quote expected standard deviations, proportions, or median survival times, we then come to a more intractable problem: the guesswork as to the effect sought. Inexperienced researchers often answer the question, "How big a difference do you want to able to detect?" with, "Any difference at all." But no sample is so large that it has a good chance of detecting the smallest conceivable difference.

One recommended approach is to choose a difference that would be clinically important—one large enough to change treatment policy. In the Venus II trial of the effect of larval therapy on healing of venous leg ulcers, researchers determined the clinically important difference in healing time by asking patients what mattered to them.[2] This is unusual, however, and more often the difference sought is the researchers' idea. An alternative is to say how big a difference the researchers think that the treatment will produce. Researchers are often wildly optimistic, and funding committees often shake their heads over the implausibility of treatment changes reducing mortality by 50% or more.

Statisticians consulted for power calculations might respond to the lack of a soundly based target difference by giving a range of sample sizes and the differences that each might detect for the researchers to ponder at leisure, but this only puts off the decision. Researchers might use this to follow an even less satisfactory path, which is to decide how many participants they can recruit, find the difference that can be detected with this sample, then claim that difference to be the one they want to find. Researchers who do this seldom describe the process in their grant applications.

In a clinical trial, we usually have more than one outcome variable of interest. If we analyse the trial using significance tests, we may carry out a large number of tests comparing the treatment groups for all these variables. Should we do a power calculation for each of them? If we test several variables, even if the treatments are identical the chance that at least one test will be significant is much higher than the nominal 0.05. To avoid this multiple testing problem, we usually identify a primary outcome variable. We need to identify this for the power calculation to design the study. Researchers often don't seem to appreciate the importance of the primary outcome variable. They change it after the study has begun, perhaps after they have seen the results of the preliminary analysis, and in many cases the original choice is not reported at all.[3] [4] This makes the reported P values invalid, over-optimistic, and potentially misleading.

Power calculations led to the call for large, simple trials,[5] [6] the first being ISIS-1.[7] This was spectacularly successful.[8] It

probably explains the 100-fold increase in sample size from 1972 to 2007.

Confidence intervals

Another reaction to the problems of small samples and of significance tests producing non-significant differences was the movement to present results in the form of confidence intervals, or bayesian credible intervals, rather than P values.[9] [10] This was motivated by the difficulties of interpreting significance tests, particularly when the result was not significant. Interval estimates for differences were seen as the best way to present the results for most types of study, particularly clinical trials, and significance tests were to be used only when an estimate was difficult or impossible. (In some situations, of course, a significance test is the better approach—when the question is primarily, "Is there any evidence?" and no meaningful estimate can be obtained.)

Many major medical journals changed their instructions to authors to say that confidence intervals would be the preferred or even required method of presentation. This was later endorsed by the wide acceptance of the CONSORT statement on the presentation of clinical trials.[11] [12] We insist on interval estimates and rightly so.

If we ask researchers to present their results as confidence intervals rather than significance tests, I think we should also ask them to base sample size calculations on confidence intervals. It is inconsistent to say that we insist on the analysis using confidence intervals but that the sample size should be decided using significance tests.

This is not difficult to do. For example, the International Carotid Stenting Study (ICSS)[13] compared the risk of stroke after angioplasty and stenting with that after surgical resection of the atheromatous plaque causing stenosis of carotid arteries. We expected that angioplasty would have a similar effect to surgery on risk reduction. The primary outcome variable was to be long term survival free of disabling stroke. There was to be an additional safety outcome of death, stroke, or myocardial infarction within 30 days and a comparison of cost. I calculated sample size based on an earlier study that reported a three year rate for ipsilateral stroke lasting more than seven days of 14%.[14] The one year rate was 11%, so most events were within the first year. There was little difference between the treatment arms. The width of the confidence interval for the difference between two similar percentages is given by observed difference $\pm 1.96\sqrt{(2p(100-p)/n)}$, where n is the number in each group and p is the percentage expected to experience the event. If we put $p=14\%$, we can calculate the confidence interval for different sample sizes (table). Similar calculations were done for other dichotomous outcomes. For health economic measures, the difference is best measured in terms of standard deviations. The width of the confidence interval is expected to be the observed difference $\pm 1.96\sigma\sqrt{(2p/n)}$, where n is the number in each treatment group and σ is the standard deviation of the economic indicator (table).

These calculations were subsequently amended slightly as outcome definitions were modified. This is the sample size account in the protocol:

The planned sample size is 1500. We do not anticipate any large difference in the principal outcome between surgery and stenting. We propose to estimate this

Sample size calculations for International Carotid Stenting Study

Total sample size	Width of 95% confidence interval	
	For estimating difference between two proportions having an event that is expected to occur in 14% of participants (% points)	For estimating difference between two means of a quantitative variable (SD)
0	±6.1	±0.18
00	±4.3	±0.12
00	±3.5	±0.10
00	±3.0	±0.09

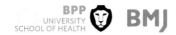

difference and present a confidence interval for difference in 30-day death, stroke or myocardial infarction and for 3-year survival free of disabling stroke or death. For 1500 patients, the 95% confidence interval will be the observed difference ±3.0 percentage points for the outcome measure of 30-day stroke, myocardial infarction and death rate and ±3.3 percentage points for the outcome measure of death or disabling stroke over 3 years of follow-up. However, the trial will have the power to detect major differences in the risks of the two procedures, for example if stenting proves to be much more risky than surgery or associated with more symptomatic restenosis. The differences detectable with a power of 80% are 4.7 percentage points for 30-day outcome and 5.1 percentage points for survival free of disabling stroke. Similar differences are detectable for secondary outcomes.[13]

Despite my best attempts, we could not exclude power calculations completely. However, the main sample size calculation was based on a confidence interval, and the study was funded.

Base sample sizes on estimation

I propose that we estimate the sample size required for clinical trials or other comparative studies by giving estimates of the likely width of the confidence interval for a set of outcome variables. This does not mean that we would not need to think about sample size; we would still have to decide whether the confidence interval was narrow enough to be worth obtaining. It does mean that we would no longer have to choose a primary outcome variable, a practice which, as noted above, is widely abused. It would have real advantages in large trials that include both clinical and economic assessment.

Power calculations have been useful. They have forced researchers to think about sample size and the likely outcome of the planned study. They have been instrumental in increasing sample sizes to levels where studies can provide much more useful information. But they have many problems, and I think it is time to leave them behind in favour of something better.

I thank Doug Altman, Martin Brown, Nicky Cullum, James Raftery, and David Torgerson for comments on an earlier draft.

Competing interests: None declared.

Provenance and peer review: Not commissioned; externally peer reviewed.

1 Cohen J. A power primer. *Psychol Bull* 1992;112:155-9.
2 Petherick ES, O'Meara S, Spilsbury K, Iglesias CP, Nelson EA, Torgerson DJ. Patient acceptability of larval therapy for leg ulcer treatment: a randomised survey to inform the sample size calculation of a randomised trial. *BMC Med Res Methodol* 2006;6:43.
3 Chan AW, Hrobjartsson A, Haahr MT, Gøtzsche PC, Altman DG. Empirical evidence for selective reporting of outcomes in randomized trials—comparison of protocols to published articles. *JAMA* 2004;291:2457-65.
4 Chan AW, Jeric K, Schmid I, Altman DG. Outcome reporting bias in randomized trials funded by the Canadian Institutes of Health Research. *CMAJ* 2004;171:735-40.
5 Peto R, Yusuf S. Need for large (but simple) trials. *Thromb Haemos* 1981;46:325.
6 Yusuf S, Collins R, Peto R. Why do we need some large, simple randomized trials? *Stat Med* 1984;3:409-20.
7 ISIS-1 (First International Study of Infarct Survival) Collaborative Group. Randomized trial of intravenous atenolol among 16 027 cases of suspected acute myocardial infarction. ISIS-I. *Lancet* 1986;ii:57-66.
8 Peto R, Collins R, Gray R. Large-scale randomized evidence: large, simple trials and overviews of trials. *J Clin Epidemiol* 1995;48:23-40.
9 Gardner MJ, Altman DG. Confidence intervals rather than P values: estimation rather than hypothesis testing. *BMJ* 1986;292:746-50.
10 Bland M. *An introduction to medical statistics* . Oxford: Oxford University Press, 1987.
11 Begg C, Cho M, Eastwood S, Horton R, Moher D, Olkin I, et al. Improving the quality of reporting of randomized controlled trials: the CONSORT statement. *JAMA* 1996;276:637-9.
12 Moher D, Schulz KF, Altman DG, CONSORT Group. The CONSORT statement: revised recommendations for improving the quality of reports of parallel-group randomised trials. *Lancet* 2001;357:1191-4
13 Featherstone RL, Brown MM, Coward LJ. International Carotid Sten Study: protocol for a randomised clinical trial comparing carotid stenting with endarterectomy in symptomatic carotid artery steno *Cerebrovasc Dis* 2004;18:69-74.
14 CAVATAS Investigators. Endovascular versus surgical treatment in patients with carotid stenosis in the Carotid and Vertebral Artery Transluminal Angioplasty Study (CAVATAS): a randomised trial. *Lan* 2001;357:1729-37.

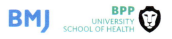

How to obtain the confidence interval from a P value

Douglas G Altman, professor of statistics in medicine[1],
Martin Bland, professor of health statistics[2]

ntre for Statistics in Medicine,
versity of Oxford, Oxford OX2

partment of Health Sciences,
versity of York, Heslington, York
o 5DD

respondence to: D G Altman
g.altman@csm.ox.ac.uk

this as: BMJ 2011;343:d2090

10.1136/bmj.d2090

://www.bmj.com/content/343/
.d2090

Confidence intervals (CIs) are widely used in reporting statistical analyses of research data, and are usually considered to be more informative than P values from significance tests.[1][2] Some published articles, however, report estimated effects and P values, but do not give CIs (a practice BMJ now strongly discourages). Here we show how to obtain the confidence interval when only the observed effect and the P value were reported.

The method is outlined in the box below in which we have distinguished two cases.

(a) Calculating the confidence interval for a difference

We consider first the analysis comparing two proportions or two means, such as in a randomised trial with a binary outcome or a measurement such as blood pressure.

For example, the abstract of a report of a randomised trial included the statement that "more patients in the zinc group than in the control group recovered by two days (49% v 32%, P=0.032)."[5] The difference in proportions was $Est = 17$ percentage points, but what is the 95% confidence interval (CI)?

Following the steps in the box we calculate the CI as follows:

$z = -0.862 + [0.743 - 2.404 \times \log(0.032)] = 2.141$;
$SE = 17/2.141 = 7.940$, so that $1.96 \times SE = 15.56$ percentage points;
95% CI is $17.0 - 15.56$ to $17.0 + 15.56$, or 1.4 to 32.6 percentage points.

(b) Calculating the confidence interval for a ratio (log transformation needed)

The calculation is trickier for ratio measures, such as risk ratio, odds ratio, and hazard ratio. We need to log transform the estimate and then reverse the procedure, as described in a previous Statistics Note.[6]

For example, the abstract of a report of a cohort study includes the statement that "In those with a [diastolic blood pressure] reading of 95-99 mm Hg the relative risk was 0.30 (P=0.034)."[7] What is the confidence interval around 0.30?

Following the steps in the box we calculate the CI as follows:

$z = -0.862 + [0.743 - 2.404 \times \log(0.034)] = 2.117$;
$Est = \log(0.30) = -1.204$;
$SE = -1.204/2.117 = -0.569$ but we ignore the minus sign, so $SE = 0.569$, and $1.96 \times SE = 1.115$;
95% CI on log scale $= -1.204 - 1.115$ to $-1.204 + 1.115 = -2.319$ to -0.089;
95% CI on natural scale $= \exp(-2.319) = 0.10$ to $\exp(-0.089) = 0.91$.

Hence the relative risk is estimated to be 0.30 with 95% CI 0.10 to 0.91.

Limitations of the method

The methods described can be applied in a wide range of settings, including the results from meta-analysis and regression analyses. The main context where they are not correct is in small samples where the outcome is continuous and the analysis has been done by a t test or analysis of variance, or the outcome is dichotomous and an exact method has been used for the confidence interval. However, even here the methods will be approximately correct in larger studies with, say, 60 patients or more.

P values presented as inequalities

Sometimes P values are very small and so are presented as P<0.0001 or something similar. The above method can be applied for small P values, setting P equal to the value it is less than, but the z statistic will be too small, hence the standard error will be too large and the resulting CI will be too wide. This is not a problem so long as we remember that the estimate is better than the interval suggests.

When we are told that P>0.05 or the difference is not significant, things are more difficult. If we apply the method described here, using P=0.05, the confidence interval will be too narrow. We must remember that the estimate is even poorer than the confidence interval calculated would suggest.

1 Gardner MJ, Altman DG. Confidence intervals rather than P values: estimation rather than hypothesis testing. BMJ 1986;292:746-50.
2 Moher D, Hopewell S, Schulz KF, Montori V, Gøtzsche PC, Devereaux PJ, et al. CONSORT 2010. Explanation and Elaboration: updated guidelines for reporting parallel group randomised trials. BMJ 2010;340:c869.
3 Lin J-T. Approximating the normal tail probability and its inverse for use on a pocket calculator. Appl Stat 1989;38:69-70.
4 Bland JM, Altman DG. Statistics Notes. Logarithms. BMJ 1996;312:700.
5 Roy SK, Hossain MJ, Khatun W, Chakraborty B, Chowdhury S, Begum A, et al. Zinc supplementation in children with cholera in Bangladesh: randomised controlled trial. BMJ 2008;336:266-8.
6 Altman DG, Bland JM. Interaction revisited: the difference between two estimates. BMJ 2003;326:219.
7 Lindblad U, Råstam L, Rydén L, Ranstam J, Isacsson S-O, Berglund G. Control of blood pressure and risk of first acute myocardial infarction: Skaraborg hypertension project. BMJ 1994;308:681.

**TEPS TO OBTAIN THE CONFIDENCE INTERVAL (CI) FOR AN ESTIMATE OF EFFECT FROM THE P VALUE
ND THE ESTIMATE (EST)**

a) CI for a difference

1 calculate the test statistic for a normal distribution test, z, from P[3]: $z = -0.862 + [0.743 - 2.404 \times \log(P)]$

2 calculate the standard error: $SE = Est/z$ (ignoring minus signs)

3 calculate the 95% CI: $Est - 1.96 \times SE$ to $Est + 1.96 \times SE$.

b) CI for a ratio

For a ratio measure, such as a risk ratio, the above formulas should be used with the estimate Est on the log scale (eg, the log risk ratio). Step 3 gives a CI on the log scale; to derive the CI on the natural scale we need to exponentiate (antilog) Est and its CI.[4]

otes

ll P values are two sided.

ll logarithms are natural (ie, to base e).[4]

or a 90% CI, we replace 1.96 by 1.65; for a 99% CI we use 2.57.

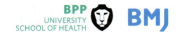

How to obtain the P value from a confidence interval

Douglas G Altman, professor of statistics in medicine[1],
J Martin Bland, professor of health statistics[2]

[1]Centre for Statistics in Medicine, University of Oxford, Oxford OX2 6UD

[2]Department of Health Sciences, University of York, Heslington, York YO10 5DD

Correspondence to: D G Altman doug.altman@csm.ox.ac.uk

Cite this as: *BMJ* 2011;343:d2304

DOI: 10.1136/bmj.d2304

http://www.bmj.com/content/343/bmj.d2304

We have shown in a previous *Statistics Note*[1] how we can calculate a confidence interval (CI) from a P value. Some published articles report confidence intervals, but do not give corresponding P values. Here we show how a confidence interval can be used to calculate a P value, should this be required. This might also be useful when the P value is given only imprecisely (eg, as P<0.05). Wherever they can be calculated, we are advocates of confidence intervals as much more useful than P values, but we like to be helpful.

The method is outlined in the box below in which we have distinguished two cases.

(a) P from CI for a difference (no transformation needed)
The simple case is when we have a CI for the difference between two means or two proportions. For example, participants in a trial received antihypertensive treatment with or without pravastatin. The authors report that pravastatin performed slightly worse than a placebo. The estimated difference between group means was 1.9 (95% CI −0.6 to 4.3) mm Hg.[4] What was the P value?

Following the steps in the box above we calculate P as follows:

$SE = [4.3 − (−0.6)]/(2×1.96) = 1.25$;
$z = 1.9/1.25 = 1.52$;
$P = \exp(−0.717×1.52 − 0.416×1.52^2) = 0.13$.

In this paper, the authors did indeed publish a P value of 0.13,[4] as we have estimated from their confidence interval.

(b) CI for a ratio (log transformation needed)
The calculation is trickier for ratio measures, such as risk ratio, odds ratio, and hazard ratio. We need to log transform the estimate and confidence limits, so that *Est*, *l*, and *u* in the box are the logarithms of the published values.

For example, in a meta-analysis of several studies comparing single versus bilateral mammary artery coronary bypass grafts Taggart et al presented a hazard ratio of 0.81, 95% CI 0.70 to 0.94.[5] They did not quote the P value.

Following the steps in the box we calculate P as follows:

$Est = \log(0.81) = −0.211$
$l = \log(0.70) = −0.357, \quad u = \log(0.94) = −0.062$
$SE = [−0.062 − (−0.357)]/(2×1.96) = 0.0753$.
$z = −0.211/0.0753 = −2.802$. We take the positive value of z, 2.802.
$P = \exp(−0.717×2.802 − 0.416×2.802^2) = 0.005$.

Limitations of the method
The formula for P is unreliable for very small P values and if your P value is smaller than 0.0001, just report it as P<0.0001.

The methods described can be applied in a wide range of settings, including the results from meta-analysis and regression analyses. The main context where they are not correct is small samples where the outcome is continuous and the analysis has been done by a *t* test or analysis of variance, or the outcome is dichotomous and an exact method has been used for the confidence interval. However, even here the methods will be approximately correct in larger studies with, say, 60 patients or more.

Contributors: JMB and DGA jointly wrote and agreed the text.

Competing interests: All authors have completed the Unified Competing Interest form at www.icmje.org/coi_disclosure.pdf (available on request from the corresponding author) and declare: support from any organisation for the submitted work; no financial relationships with any organisations that might have an interest in the submitted work in the previous 3 years; no other relationships or activities that could appear to have influenced the submitted work.

1 Altman DG, Bland JM. How to obtain a confidence interval from a P value. *BMJ* 2011;342:d2090.
2 Lin J-T. Approximating the normal tail probability and its inverse for use on a pocket calculator. *Appl Stat* 1989;38:69-70.
3 Mancia G, Parati G, Revera M, Bilo G, Giuliano A, Veglia F, et al. Statin antihypertensive treatment, and blood pressure control in clinic and over 24 hours: evidence from PHYLLIS randomised double blind trial. *BMJ* 2010;340:c1197.
4 Taggart DP, D'Amico R, Altman DG. Effect of arterial revascularisation on survival: a systematic review of studies comparing bilateral and single internal mammary arteries. *Lancet* 2001;358:870-5.
5 Bland JM, Altman DG. Logarithms. *BMJ* 1996;312:700.

STEPS TO OBTAIN THE P VALUE FROM THE CI FOR AN ESTIMATE OF EFFECT (*EST*)

(a) P from CI for a difference

If the upper and lower limits of a 95% CI are *u* and *l* respectively:

1 calculate the standard error: $SE = (u − l)/(2×1.96)$
2 calculate the test statistic: $z = Est/SE$
3 calculate the P value[2]: $P = \exp(−0.717×z − 0.416×z^2)$.

(b) P from CI for a ratio

For a ratio measure, such as a risk ratio, the above formulas should be used with the estimate *Est* and the confidence limits on the log scale (eg, the log risk ratio and its CI).

Notes
All P values are two sided.
All logarithms are natural (ie, to base e).[3]
"exp" is the exponential function.
The formula for P works only for positive z, so if z is negative we remove the minus sign.
For a 90% CI, we replace 1.96 by 1.65; for a 99% CI we use 2.57.

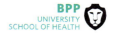

Clinicians are right not to like Cohen's κ

Henrica C W de Vet, professor of clinimetrics[1], Lidwine B Mokkink, junior researcher of clinimetrics[1], Caroline B Terwee, assistant professor of clinimetrics[1], Otto S Hoekstra, professor of nuclear medicine[2], Dirk L Knol, assistant professor of statistics[1]

artment of Epidemiology
Biostatistics, EMGO Institute
ealth and Care Research,
Iniversity Medical Center,
terdam, Netherlands

artment of Radiology and
ear Medicine, VU University
ical Center, Amsterdam,
erlands

espondence to: H C W de Vet
devet@vumc.nl

this as: *BMJ* 2013;346:f2125

10.1136/bmj.f2125

//www.bmj.com/content/346/
f2125

Introduction

Observer variation is the Achilles' heel in clinical diagnoses such as medical imaging.[1] It directly affects the value of diagnostic tests and other measurements in clinical practice. Clinicians interested in observer variation pose questions such as "Is my diagnosis in agreement with that of my colleagues?" (interobserver) and "Would I obtain the same result if I repeated the assessment?" (intraobserver). To express the level of intraobserver or interobserver agreement, many epidemiology and medical statistics textbooks[2] [3] recommend Cohen's κ as the most adequate measure. Cohen introduced κ as a coefficient of agreement for categorical outcomes.[4] Clinicians and researchers, however, have long been unhappy with κ because a high level of agreement can be accompanied by a low κ value. These counterintuitive results have led to dissatisfaction with κ expressed in papers with titles containing terms such as "paradox" and "bias" and calling for extensions and adjustments of κ.[5] [6]

An example of a confusing situation is provided by Bruynesteyn and colleagues in a study on rheumatoid arthritis that examined progression of joint damage based on pairs of radiographs from 46 patients.[7] The authors compared the interobserver agreement between rheumatologists in two situations: firstly, when the pairs of radiographs were assessed in a chronological order and, secondly, when the rheumatologists had no knowledge about the order (random order). Table 1 shows the proportion of observed agreement and the value of κ for these two situations.

The highest value for the proportion of observed agreement was seen in the "chronological order" set, yet the highest κ value was seen in the "random order" set. The conclusion about which situation is preferred is therefore unclear.

In this paper we will first show how κ is calculated and explain these seemingly contradictory results. We will show how κ is a relative measure of observer variation, whereas the questions posed by clinicians require an absolute measure of agreement. Finally, we will focus on absolute measures of agreement.

ABSTRACT

Clinicians are interested in observer variation in terms of the probability of other raters (interobserver) or themselves (intraobserver) obtaining the same answer. Cohen's κ is commonly used in the medical literature to express such agreement in categorical outcomes. The value of Cohen's κ, however, is not sufficiently informative because it is a relative measure, while the clinician's question of observer variation calls for an absolute measure. Using an example in which the observed agreement and κ lead to different conclusions, we illustrate that percentage agreement is an absolute measure (a measure of agreement) and that κ is a relative measure (a measure of reliability).

For the data to be useful for clinicians, measures of agreement should be used. The proportion of specific agreement, expressing the agreement separately for the positive and the negative ratings, is the most appropriate measure for conveying the relevant information in a 2×2 table and is most informative for clinicians.

Calculation of Cohen's κ

In their paper, Bruynesteyn and colleagues[7] did not provide the raw data for the 2×2 tables. This gives us the opportunity to come up with numbers that mimic their results but are more attractive from an educational viewpoint. The first example presented by Bruynestein and colleagues might have resembled the data in table 2.

The two rheumatologists, A and B, agree with each other on 38 out of the 46 sets of radiographs: in 33 cases they both observe progression and in five cases they both observe no progression. Therefore, the proportion of observed agreement (P_o) is $(a+d)/N=(33+5)/46=0.826$. Part of the observed agreement between two raters, however, is attributable to chance. As with multiple choice questions in an exam, some questions are answered correctly simply by guessing. Thus, in some cases, rheumatologist B might have agreed with rheumatologist A just by chance, even if neither of them had looked carefully at the radiographs. This is called "agreement by chance" or "expected agreement" (P_e). Cohen's κ adjusts for this expected agreement.[4] Multiplying the row and column totals corresponding to each cell and dividing by the grand total (N) provides the expected agreement for each cell in case of independent judgments. Therefore, the expected agreement in cell a is $(37×37)/46=29.76$ cases, while the expected agreement in cell d is $(9×9)/46=1.76$ cases. Consequently, the total proportion of expected agreement (P_e) amounts to $(29.76+1.76)/46=0.685$.

The formula for Cohen's κ is $(P_o-P_e)/(1-P_e)$. In the numerator, the expected agreement is subtracted from the observed agreement. The denominator is also adjusted for the expected agreement. In this example, $P_o=0.826$ and $P_e=0.685$. Filling in the formula yields $κ=(0.826-0.685)/(1-0.685)=0.45$.

SUMMARY POINTS

- As Cohens's κ was originally introduced as a coefficient of agreement for categorical variables, researchers often use Cohen's κ to express observer agreement in clinical diagnoses

- Cohen's κ is falsely known as an agreement measure, whereas it is a measure of reliability. Agreement measures are absolute measures, and reliability measures are relative measures relating the absolute agreement or measurement error of a characteristic to its variation in the sample

- The proportion of specific agreement, rather than Cohen's κ, is an informative agreement measure for clinicians

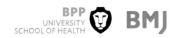

Table 1 Observed agreement and κ values for "chronological order" and "random order" sets (adapted from Bruynesteyn et al[7])

	Prevalence of progression of joint damage	Observed agreement (proportion)	Cohen's κ
Chronological order	80%	0.85	0.45
Random order	37%	0.80	0.60

Table 2 Example 1: 2×2 table of "chronological order" dataset

		Rheumatologist A		
Rheumatologist B	Progression	No progression	Total	
Progression	33 (a)	4 (b)	37	
No progression	4 (c)	5 (d)	9	
Total	37	9	46 (N)	

Table 3 Example 2: 2×2 table of "random order" dataset

		Rheumatologist A		
Rheumatologist B	Progression	No progression	Total	
Progression	13 (a)	3 (b)	16	
No progression	5 (c)	25 (d)	30	
Total	18	28	46 (N)	

BOX 1 FORMULA AND INTERPRETATION OF A RELIABILITY MEASURE

The formula for a reliability measure (Rel) of continuous outcomes is:

$$Rel = (\sigma^2 p)/(\sigma^2 p + \sigma^2 error)$$

A reliability measure relates the measurement error variance ($\sigma^2 error$) to the variability between people ($\sigma^2 p$). In this formula, $\sigma^2 error$ represents how close the scores of repeated assessments are. The square root of $\sigma^2 error$ equals the standard error of measurement, which is expressed in the units of measurement—for example, 0.5 kg in case of weighing scales. When measuring body weight in adults, $\sigma^2 error$ will be small compared with the variation in the sample ($\sigma^2 p$), and the reliability measure will be close to 1 (excellent reliability), but when $\sigma^2 error$ is large compared with the variation in the sample (for example, when measuring birth weight) the reliability measure will be closer to 0 (poor reliability).

Example 2 mimics the situation in which the two rheumatologists have examined the 46 radiographs in "random order." The results of the 2×2 table might have resembled the data in table 3.

In the second example 2 (table 3), we once again observe an agreement of 0.826 ((13+25)/46). The expected agreement is now (18×16)/46=6.26 for "progression" and (28×30)/46=18.26 for "no progression." This amounts to a proportion of 0.533 ((6.26+18.26)/46) for expected agreement. The resulting κ value is (0.826−0.533)/(1−0.533)=0.63.

Example 2 shows the same proportion of observed agreement as example 1 (38/46 in both cases), but Cohen's κ value is higher. This is because of the difference in expected agreement. The row and column totals of the 2×2 table can be seen as the prevalence of progression, as observed by the two rheumatologists. The observed prevalence of progression was 80% (37/46) in example 1 and only 37% (17/46) in example 2 (averaged over two raters). The expected agreement is particularly high when the prevalence of abnormalities is either very high or very low (the prevalence of progression is 80% in example 1). It is in these situations that a high proportion of agreement can result in a low value of κ.

These examples show that a lower κ value is caused by higher expected agreement (as in example 1). It is still unclear, however, whether researchers should rely on the proportion of observed agreement or the κ value. To answer this question, we will first elaborate on relative and absolute measures of agreement.

Absolute and relative measures to quantify observer variation

Agreement represents an absolute measure and reliabilit a relative measure (box 1 shows the formula and statist details).[8][9] The difference between agreement and reliab is most easily explained for situations of continu outcomes, such as body weight. When a person's b weight is measured by different raters, we are interes in how much the observed weights differ. This is absolute measure of variation—called the measurem error or extent of agreement—and can be expressed units of measurement, such as kilograms. We want measurement error to be as small as possible. Reliabi is a relative measure as it relates the measurement e to the variation within a study sample. If the measurem error is small compared with the variation within sample, the reliability is high. In a sample of adults, b weight varies from about 50 kg to more than 100 kg. variation is much larger than that seen in birth wei which might range from about 1.5 to 5 kg. Thus, babies f a more homogeneous sample than adults and there a measurement error of 0.5 kg in measurement of b weight will lead to lower reliability. Consequently, weigh scales with this degree of error would not be suitable measure birth weight.

Categorical outcomes, on the other hand, are based o on classifications and have no units of measurement. these situations, closeness of the scores and measurem error are expressed as the probability of misclassificati or the proportion of observed agreement. The relat measure for categorical variables is Cohen's κ.

Cohen's κ is a reliability measure

Cohen's κ is a relative measure[9] because it relates proportion of observed agreement (the absolute measu to variation in the sample and corresponds with a spec type of reliability measure.[10] At this point, it is import to explain how variation is assessed in a sample w categorical or even dichotomous variables. In case categorical outcomes, the sample is homogeneous all patients have the same outcome (that is, are in same category). A sample is maximally heterogene if the patients are equally distributed over the exist categories (that is, in case of dichotomous outcome 50-50 distribution). So, the row and column totals of 2×2 table—that is, the prevalence of abnormalities normalities—give an indication of the heterogeneity of sample. In case of a prevalence of 50% (50-50 distributio the expected agreement will be minimal. With a higher lower prevalence—that is, a more skewed distribution— expected agreement will be greater and, assuming the sa proportion of observed agreement, the value of κ will smaller. This explains the findings in examples 1 and (tables 2 and 3): while the absolute agreement is the sar the value of κ (as a relative measure) is lower in exam 1 because the distribution of progression in the sample more skewed.

So, whether we should rely on Cohen's κ or on a meas of agreement now comes down to whether the clini question concerns reliability or agreement.

Do clinical questions concern reliability or agreement?

In clinical practice, clinicians perform assessments diagnose and monitor individual patients. They pe questions regarding observer variation such as "Will

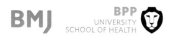

diagnosis be in agreement with a colleague's diagnosis?" and "Can I distinguish patients with abnormal scores from those with normal scores?" The first question clearly concerns agreement and requires an absolute measure of agreement. Thus, in a situation of continuous outcomes, such as body weight, the clinicians would want to know how close the observed weights were in terms of absolute difference in the units of measurement, and, in case of categorical variables such as radiological classifications, they would want to know the probability of agreement.

When clinicians ask whether patients with abnormal scores can be distinguished from those with normal scores, they also have individual patients in mind and are not considering the distribution of a sample of patients. This is illustrated by the radiological assessment of progression in patients with rheumatoid arthritis (tables 2 and 3). We see that the prevalence of progression is higher when rheumatologists judge the radiographs in chronological order rather than in random order (80% v 37%). They more often observe "progression," which means that they tend to label smaller differences as progression in the chronological order set. The observed agreement between the two observers is the same, but the relative measure is lower because the distribution is more skewed. Thus, taking the sample distribution into account results in a relative measure, which is not what clinicians have in mind when they ask whether they can distinguish between people with abnormal and normal scores.

Reliability is at stake if we want to know whether a specific test is suitable for identifying or classifying patients in a certain sample. For example, in the case of screening the underlying question is: "Can we identify patients with abnormalities in a large population sample?" Another reliability question concerns the evaluation of a new classification system for a test or measurement instrument: one might question whether raters can distinguish between the proposed categories. These issues involve the ability to distinguish between patients in population samples. Thus, when variation within the sample is of interest, reliability measures are preferred. This is the case when the research question refers to suitability of a test in a particular setting. In clinical practice, clinicians are interested in decision making in individual patients and therefore absolute measures are of interest.

Proportion of specific agreement as preferred measure of agreement

If rheumatologists have to decide which measure they would prefer to use to rate progression, they should consider an absolute measure of agreement as κ fails to provide any information that would help them interpret the results for their patients in clinical practice.

One such measure could be the proportion of observed agreement. The question, however, is whether this measure is sufficiently informative. The best information is provided by the complete 2×2 table itself. In table 2, the problem of misclassification seems to be most marked in the case of "no progression," where the numbers on which the rheumatologists disagree (cells b and c) outweigh the numbers on which they do agree (cell d). On the other hand, there is no problem with the classification of "progression" (cell a versus cells b and c). This dual information cannot be captured in a single statistic and therefore the proportion of observed agreement is not sufficiently informative either. The measure that would convey this information best is the proportion of specific agreement. This is a measure

that expresses the agreement separately for positive and negative ratings—that is, agreement on the diagnosis of "progression" and on the diagnosis of "no progression." The specific agreement on a positive rating, known as the positive agreement, is calculated by the following formula[11]: $PA=2a/(2a+b+c)$, while specific agreement on a negative rating, the negative agreement, is calculated using the formula: $NA=2d/(2d+b+c)$. The inclusion of both cells b and c in the formula accounts for the fact that these numbers might be different (see table 3), and therefore their mean value is taken.

The proportion of specific agreement helps the clinician answer questions such as: "Suppose I rate 'progression' based on a pair of radiographs, what is the probability that another clinician would also rate 'progression'?" In the case of example 1 (table 2), where the observed prevalence of progression was 80%, the answer would be $PA=(2\times33)/((2\times33)+4+4)=0.892$—that is, 89.2% for agreement on "progression"—and $NA=(2\times5)/((2\times5)+4+4)=0.556$—that is, 55.6% for agreement on "no progression."

In the case of example 2 (table 3), where the prevalence of progression was 37%, the probability that other clinicians would also observe progression would be $PA=(2\times13)/((2\times13)+3+5)=0.765$—that is, 76.5% for "progression"—and $NA=(2\times25)/((2\times25)+3+5)=0.862$—that is, 86.2% for "no progression."

Note that in the above formulas the same numbers of disagreements (that is, cells b and c) are related to the agreements on the positive ratings (cell a) and to the agreements on the negative ratings (cell d). We see again the influence of prevalence, but now it has direct clinical meaning as it is transformed into a probability of agreement for positive and negative ratings. When a sample is homogeneous because almost all patients show progression (example 1), the probability of observer agreement on progression is higher. Similarly, when only a small number of patients have no progression, the probability of observer agreement on non-progression becomes smaller, despite the same numbers of misclassification. Consequently, the proportion of specific agreement corresponds better with the reasoning of a clinician. Moreover, distinguishing between the proportion of agreement for positive and negative ratings makes sense because both outcomes have different clinical consequences.

It is interesting to note that the measure of specific agreement was first described by Dice in 1945[11] and later revitalised in the medical literature by Cicchetti and Feinstein.[12] Until now, however, it has not found broad application, despite being an extremely helpful measure for clinicians.

Conclusion

As a mnemonic, clinicians might like to remember that Agreement is an Absolute measure and that RELiability is a RELative measure to quantify observer variation. Cohen introduced κ as a measure of agreement and many authors have followed suit as the need to take chance agreement into account sounds quite plausible. Adjustment of the observed agreement for the expected agreement, however, turns κ into a relative measure. Therefore, we should stop adapting Cohen's κ and instead be critical about whether a specific clinical question asks for a measure of reliability or a measure of agreement. In particular, Cohen's κ is not to be recommended as a measure of observer variation in clinical practice. Such questions regarding a clinician's confidence in a specific diagnosis concern agreement and, as such,

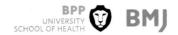

require an absolute measure of agreement. The measure of specific agreement best conveys the relevant information contained in a 2×2 table and is most helpful for clinical practice.

Contributors: All authors had a substantial contribution to the conception and design of the paper. HCWdV drafted the paper, and all other authors added intellectual content and critically reviewed and revised the paper. All authors have approved the final version. HCWdV is guarantor.

Competing interests: All authors have completed the ICMJE uniform disclosure form at www.icmje.org/coi_disclosure.pdf (available on request from the corresponding author) and declare: no support from any organisation for the submitted work; no financial relationships with any organisations that might have an interest in the submitted work in the previous three years; no other relationships or activities that could appear to have influenced the submitted work.

Provenance and peer review: Not commissioned; externally peer reviewed.

1   Robinson PJ. Radiology's Achilles' heel: error and variation in the interpretation of the Röntgen image. *Br J Radiol* 1997;70:1085-98
2   Sackett D, Haynes RB, Guyatt GH, Tugwell P. Clinical epidemiology—a basic science for clinical medicine. Little, Brown and Company, 1991:25-31.
3   Altman DG. Practical statistics for medical research. Chapman and Hall/CRC Press, 1991:403-9.
4   Cohen J. A coefficient of agreement for nominal scales. *Educational and Psychological Measurement* 1960;20:37-46.
5   Feinstein AR, Cicchetti DV. High agreement but low kappa: I. the problems of two paradoxes. *J Clin Epidemiol* 1990;43:543-9.
6   Byrt T, Bishop J, Carlin JB. Bias, prevalence and kappa. *J Clin Epidemiol* 1993;46:423-9.
7   Bruynesteyn K, Van Der Heijde D, Boers M, Saudan A, Peloso P, Paulus H, et al. Detecting radiological changes in rheumatoid arthritis that are considered important by clinical experts: influence of reading with or without known sequence. *J Rheumatol* 2002;29:2306-12.
8   De Vet HCW, Terwee CB, Knol DL, Bouter LM. When to use agreement versus reliability measures. *J Clin Epidemiol* 2006;59:1033-9.
9   Kottner J, Audigé L, Brorson S, Donner A, Gajewski BJ, Hrobjartsson A, et al. Guidelines for reporting reliability and agreement studies (GRRAS) were proposed. *J Clin Epidemiol* 2011;64:96-106.
10 Fleiss JL, Cohen J. The equivalence of weighted kappa and the intraclass correlation coefficient as measures of reliability. *Educational and Psychological Measurement* 1973;33:613-9.
11 Dice LR. Measures of the amount of ecologic association between species. *Ecology* 1945;26:297-302.
12 Cicchetti DV, Feinstein AR. High agreement but low kappa: II Resolving the paradoxes. *J Clin Epidemiol* 1990;43:551-8.

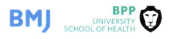

The Cochrane Collaboration's tool for assessing risk of bias in randomised trials

Julian P T Higgins, senior statistician[1], Douglas G Altman, director[2], Peter C Gøtzsche, director[3], Peter Jüni, head of division[4], David Moher, senior scientist[5][6], Andrew D Oxman, senior researcher[7], Jelena Savović, postdoctoral fellow[8], Kenneth F Schulz, vice president[9], Laura Weeks, research associate[5], Jonathan A C Sterne, professor of medical statistics and epidemiology[8], Cochrane Bias Methods Group, Cochrane Statistical Methods Group

Biostatistics Unit, Institute
blic Health, Cambridge CB2
UK

tre for Statistics in Medicine,
ersity of Oxford, Oxford, UK

Nordic Cochrane Centre,
ospitalet and University of
nhagen, Denmark

tute of Social and Preventive
icine, University of Bern,
zerland

artment of Epidemiology and
munity Medincine, Faculty of
icine, University of Ottawa,
da

artment of Epidemiology and
munity Medicine, Faculty of
icine, University of Ottawa,
da

entive and International
th Care Unit, Norwegian
wledge Centre for the Health
ices, Oslo, Norway

artment of Social Medicine,
ersity of Bristol, Bristol, UK

Research Triangle Park, North
lina, USA

espondence to: J P T Higgins
n.higgins@mrc-bsu.cam.ac.uk.

this as: BMJ 2011;343:d5928

10.1136/bmj.d5928

://www.bmj.com/content/343/
d5928

Randomised trials, and systematic reviews of such trials, provide the most reliable evidence about the effects of healthcare interventions. Provided that there are enough participants, randomisation should ensure that participants in the intervention and comparison groups are similar with respect to both known and unknown prognostic factors. Differences in outcomes of interest between the different groups can then in principle be ascribed to the causal effect of the intervention.[1]

Causal inferences from randomised trials can, however, be undermined by flaws in design, conduct, analyses, and reporting, leading to underestimation or overestimation of the true intervention effect (bias).[2] However, it is usually impossible to know the extent to which biases have affected the results of a particular trial.

Systematic reviews aim to collate and synthesise all studies that meet prespecified eligibility criteria[3] using methods that attempt to minimise bias. To obtain reliable conclusions, review authors must carefully consider the potential limitations of the included studies. The notion of study "quality" is not well defined but relates to the extent to which its design, conduct, analysis, and presentation were appropriate to answer its research question. Many tools for assessing the quality of randomised trials are available, including scales (which score the trials) and checklists (which assess trials without producing a score).[4][5][6][7] Until recently, Cochrane reviews used a variety of these tools, mainly checklists.[8] In 2005 the Cochrane Collaboration's methods groups embarked on a new strategy for assessing the quality of randomised trials. In this paper we describe the collaboration's new risk of bias assessment tool, and the process by which it was developed and evaluated.

Development of risk assessment tool

In May 2005, 16 statisticians, epidemiologists, and review authors attended a three day meeting to develop the new tool. Before the meeting, JPTH and DGA compiled an extensive list of potential sources of bias in clinical trials. The items on the list were divided into seven areas: generation of the allocation sequence; concealment of the

ABSTRACT

Flaws in the design, conduct, analysis, and reporting of randomised trials can cause the effect of an intervention to be underestimated or overestimated. The Cochrane Collaboration's tool for assessing risk of bias aims to make the process clearer and more accurate

allocation sequence; blinding; attrition and exclusions; other generic sources of bias; biases specific to the trial design (such as crossover or cluster randomised trials); and biases that might be specific to a clinical specialty. For each of the seven areas, a nominated meeting participant prepared a review of the empirical evidence, a discussion of specific issues and uncertainties, and a proposed set of criteria for assessing protection from bias as adequate, inadequate, or unclear, supported by examples.

During the meeting decisions were made by informal consensus regarding items that were truly potential biases rather than sources of heterogeneity or imprecision. Potential biases were then divided into domains, and strategies for their assessment were agreed, again by informal consensus, leading to the creation of a new tool for assessing potential for bias. Meeting participants also discussed how to summarise assessments across domains, how to illustrate assessments, and how to incorporate assessments into analyses and conclusions. Minutes of the meeting were transcribed from an audio recording in conjunction with written notes.

After the meeting, pairs of authors developed detailed criteria for each included item in the tool and guidance for assessing the potential for bias. Documents were shared and feedback requested from the whole working group (including six who could not attend the meeting). Several email iterations took place, which also incorporated feedback from presentations of the proposed guidance at various meetings and workshops within the Cochrane Collaboration and from pilot work by selected review teams in collaboration with members of the working group. The materials were integrated by the co-leads into comprehensive guidance on the new risk of bias tool. This was published in February 2008 and adopted as the recommended method throughout the Cochrane Collaboration.[9]

Evaluation phase

A three stage project to evaluate the tool was initiated in early 2009. A series of focus groups was held in which review authors who had used the tool were asked to reflect on their experiences. Findings from the focus groups were then fed into the design of questionnaires for use in three online surveys of review authors who had used the tool, review

SUMMARY POINTS

- Systematic reviews should carefully consider the potential limitations of the studies included
- The Cochrane Collaboration has developed a new tool for assessing risk of bias in randomised trials
- The tool separates a judgment about risk of bias from a description of the support for that judgment, for a series of items covering different domains of bias

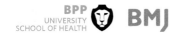

authors who had not used the tool (to explore why not), and editorial teams within the collaboration. We held a meeting to discuss the findings from the focus groups and surveys and to consider revisions to the first version of the risk of bias tool. This was attended by six participants from the 2005 meeting and 17 others, including statisticians, epidemiologists, coordinating editors and other staff of Cochrane review groups, and the editor in chief of the *Cochrane Library*.

The risk of bias tool

At the 2005 workshop the participants agreed the seven principles on which the new risk of bias assessment tool was based (box).

The risk of bias tool covers six domains of bias: selection bias, performance bias, detection bias, attrition bias, reporting bias, and other bias. Within each domain, assessments are made for one or more items, which may cover different aspects of the domain, or different outcomes. Table 1 shows the recommended list of items. These are discussed in more detail in the appendix on bmj.com.

For each item in the tool, the assessment of risk of bias i two parts. The support for judgment provides a succinct text description or summary of the relevant trial characteri on which judgments of risk of bias are based and aim ensure transparency in how judgments are reached. example, the item about concealment of the random allocation sequence would provide details of what meas were in place, if any, to conceal the sequence. Information these descriptions will often come from a single publis trial report but may be obtained from a mixture of reports, protocols, published comments on the trial, contacts with the investigators. The support for the judgm should provide a summary of known facts, including verba quotes where possible. The source of this information sh be stated, and when there is no information on which to b a judgment, this should be stated.

The second part of the tool involves assigning a judgm of high, low, or unclear risk of material bias for each item. define material bias as bias of sufficient magnitude to h a notable effect on the results or conclusions of the tr

---

PRINCIPLES FOR ASSESSING RISK OF BIAS

1. Do not use quality scales
Quality scales and resulting scores are not an appropriate way to appraise clinical trials. They tend to combine assessments of aspects of the quality of reporting with aspects of trial conduct, and to assign weights to different items in ways that are difficult to justify. Both theoretical considerations[10] and empirical evidence[11] suggest that associations of different scales with intervention effec estimates are inconsistent and unpredictable

2. Focus on internal validity
The internal validity of a study is the extent to which it is free from bias. It is important to separate assessment of internal validity from that of external validity (generalisability or applicability) and precision (the extent to which study results are free from random error). Applicability depends on the purpose for which the study is to be used and is less relevant without internal validity. Precisio depends on the number of participants and events in a study. A small trial with low risk of bias may provide very imprecise results with a wide confidence interval. Conversely, the results of a large trial may be precise (narrow confidence interval) but have a high risk of bias if internal validity is poor

3. Assess the risk of bias in trial results, not the quality of reporting or methodological problems that are not directly related to risk of bias
The quality of reporting, such as whether details were described or not, affects the ability of systematic review authors and users of medical research to assess the risk of bias but is not directly related to the risk of bias. Similarly, some aspects of trial conduct, such as obtaining ethical approval or calculating sample size, are not directly related to the risk of bias. Conversely, results of a tria that used the best possible methods may still be at risk of bias. For example, blinding may not be feasible in many non-drug trials, and it would not be reasonable to consider the trial as low quality because of the absence of blinding. Nonetheless, many types of outcome may be influenced by participants' knowledge of the intervention received, and so the trial results for such outcomes may be considered to be at risk of bias because of the absence of blinding, despite this being impossible to achieve

4. Assessments of risk of bias require judgment
Assessment of whether a particular aspect of trial conduct renders its results at risk of bias requires both knowledge of the trial methods and a judgment about whether those methods are likely to have led to a risk of bias. We decided that the basis for bias assessments should be made explicit, by recording the aspects of the trial methods on which the judgment was based and then th judgment itself

5. Choose domains to be assessed based on a combination of theoretical and empirical considerations
Empirical studies show that particular aspects of trial conduct are associated with bias.[2] [12] However, these studies did not include al potential sources of bias. For example, available evidence does not distinguish between different aspects of blinding (of participants health professionals, and outcome assessment) and is very limited with regard to how authors dealt with incomplete outcome data. There may also be topic specific and design specific issues that are relevant only to some trials and reviews. For example, in a review containing crossover trials it might be appropriate to assess whether results were at risk of bias because there was an insufficient "washout" period between the two treatment periods

6. Focus on risk of bias in the data as represented in the review rather than as originally reported
Some papers may report trial results that are considered as at high risk of bias, for which it may be possible to derive a result at lo risk of bias. For example, a paper that inappropriately excluded certain patients from analyses might report the intervention groups and outcomes for these patients, so that the omitted participants can be reinstated

7. Report outcome specific evaluations of risk of bias
Some aspects of trial conduct (for example, whether the randomised allocation was concealed at the time the participant was recruited) apply to the trial as a whole. For other aspects, however, the risk of bias is inherently specific to different outcomes within the trial. For example, all cause mortality might be ascertained through linkages to death registries (low risk of bias), while recurrence of cancer might have been assessed by a doctor with knowledge of the allocated intervention (high risk of bias

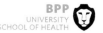

Table 1 Cochrane Collaboration's tool for assessing risk of bias (adapted from Higgins and ...man[13])

...as domain	Source of bias	Support for judgment	Review authors' judgment (assess as low, unclear or high risk of bias)
...lection bias	Random sequence generation	Describe the method used to generate the allocation sequence in sufficient detail to allow an assessment of whether it should produce comparable groups	Selection bias (biased allocation to interventions) due to inadequate generation of a randomised sequence
	Allocation concealment	Describe the method used to conceal the allocation sequence in sufficient detail to determine whether intervention allocations could have been foreseen before or during enrolment	Selection bias (biased allocation to interventions) due to inadequate concealment of allocations before assignment
...rformance bias	Binding of participants and personnel*	Describe all measures used, if any, to blind trial participants and researchers from knowledge of which intervention a participant received. Provide any information relating to whether the intended blinding was effective	Performance bias due to knowledge of the allocated interventions by participants and personnel during the study
...tection bias	Blinding of outcome assessment*	Describe all measures used, if any, to blind outcome assessment from knowledge of which intervention a participant received. Provide any information relating to whether the intended blinding was effective	Detection bias due to knowledge of the allocated interventions by outcome assessment
...trition bias	Incomplete outcome data*	Describe the completeness of outcome data for each main outcome, including attrition and exclusions from the analysis. State whether attrition and exclusions were reported, the numbers in each intervention group (compared with total randomised participants), reasons for attrition or exclusions where reported, and any reinclusions in analyses for the review	Attrition bias due to amount, nature, or handling of incomplete outcome data
...porting bias	selective reporting	State how selective outcome reporting was examined and what was found	Reporting bias due to selective outcome reporting
...her bias	Anything else, ideally prespecified	State any important concerns about bias not covered in the other domains in the tool	Bias due to problems not covered elsewhere

*...sessments should be made for each main outcome or class of outcomes.

recognising the subjectivity of any such judgment. Detailed criteria for making judgments about the risk of bias from each of the items in the tool are available in the *Cochrane Handbook*.[13] If insufficient detail is reported of what happened in the trial, the judgment will usually be unclear risk of bias. A judgment of unclear risk should also be made if what happened in the trial is known but the associated risk of bias is unknown—for example, if participants take additional drugs of unknown effectiveness as a result of them being aware of their intervention assignment. We recommend that judgments be made independently by at least two people, with any discrepancies resolved by discussion in the first instance.

Some of the items in the tool, such as methods for randomisation, require only a single assessment for each trial included in the review. For other items, such as blinding and incomplete outcome data, two or more assessments may be used because they generally need to be made separately for different outcomes (or for the same outcome at different time points). However, we recommend that review authors limit the number of assessments used by grouping outcomes—for example, as subjective or objective for the purposes of assessing blinding of outcome assessment or as "patient reported at 6 months" or "patient reported at 12 months" for assessing risk of bias due to incomplete outcome data.

Evaluation of initial implementation
The first (2008) version of the tool was slightly different from the one we present here. The 2008 version did not categorise biases by the six domains (selection bias, performance bias, etc); had a single assessment for blinding; and expressed risk of bias in the format '"yes," "no," or "unclear" (referring to lack of a risk) rather than as low, high, or unclear risk. The 2010 evaluation of the initial version found wide acceptance of the need for the risk of bias tool, with a consensus that it represents an improvement over methods previously recommended by the Collaboration or widely used in systematic reviews.

Participants in the focus groups noted that the tool took longer to complete than previous methods. Of 187 authors surveyed, 88% took longer than 10 minutes to complete the new tool, 44% longer than 20 minutes, and 7% longer than an hour, but 83% considered the time taken acceptable. There was consensus that classifying items in the tool according to categories of bias (selection bias, performance bias, etc) would help users, so we introduced these. There was also consensus that assessment of blinding should be separated into blinding of participants and health professionals (performance bias) and blinding of outcome assessment (detection bias) and that the phrasing of the judgments about risk should be changed to low, high, and unclear risk. The domains reported to be the most difficult to assess were risk of bias due to incomplete outcome data and selective reporting of outcomes. There was agreement that improved training materials and availability of worked examples would increase the quality and reliability of bias assessments.

Presentation of assessments
Results of an assessment of risk of bias can be presented in a table, in which judgments for each item in each trial are presented alongside their descriptive justification. Table 2 presents an example of a risk of bias table for one trial included in a Cochrane review of therapeutic monitoring of antiretrovirals for people with HIV.[14] Risks of bias due to blinding and incomplete outcome data were assessed across all outcomes within each included study, rather than separately for different outcomes as will be more appropriate in some situations.

Presenting risk of bias tables for every study in a review can be cumbersome, and we suggest that illustrations are used to summarise the judgments in the main systematic review document. The figure provides an example. Here the judgments apply to all meta-analyses in the review. An alternative would be to illustrate the risk of bias for a particular meta-analysis (or for a particular outcome if a statistical synthesis is not undertaken), showing the proportion of information that comes from studies at low,

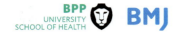

Table 2 Example of risk of bias table from a Cochrane review[14]

Bias	Authors' judgment	Support for judgment
Random sequence generation (selection bias)	Low risk	Quote: "Randomization was one to one with a block of size 6. The list of randomization was obtained using the SAS procedure plan at the data statistical analysis centre"
Allocation concealment (selection bias)	Unclear risk	The randomisation list was created at the statistical data centre, but further description of allocation is not included
Blinding of participants and researchers (performance bias)	High risk	Open label
Incomplete outcome data (attrition bias)	Low risk	Losses to follow-up were disclosed and the analyses were conducted using, firstly, a modified intention to treat analysis in which missing=failures and, secondly, on an observed basis. Although the authors describe an intention to treat analysis, the 139 participants initially randomised were not all included; five were excluded (four withdrew and one had lung cancer diagnosed). This is a reasonable attrition and not expected to affect results. Adequate sample size of 60 per group was achieved
Selective reporting (reporting bias)	Low risk	All prespecified outcomes were reported
Other bias	Unclear risk	No description of the uptake of the therapeutic drug monitoring recommendations by physicians, which could result in performance bias

Table 3 Approach to formulating summary assessments of risk of bias for each important outcome (across domains) within and across trials (adapted from Higgins and Altman[13])

Risk of bias	Interpretation	Within a trial	Across trials
Low risk of bias	Bias, if present, is unlikely to alter the results seriously	Low risk of bias for all key domains	Most information is from trials at low risk of bias
Unclear risk of bias	A risk of bias that raises some doubt about the results	Low or unclear risk of bias for all key domains	Most information is from trials at low or unclear risk of bias
High risk of bias	Bias may alter the results seriously	High risk of bias for one or more key domains	The proportion of information from trials at high risk of bias is sufficient to affect the interpretation of results

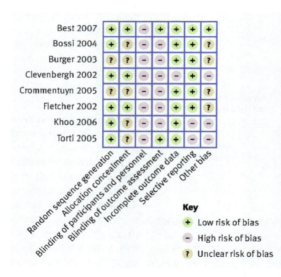

Fig 1 Example presentation of risk of bias assessments for studies in a Cochrane review of therapeutic monitoring of antiretroviral drugs in people with HIV[14]

unclear, or high risk of bias for each item in the tool, among studies contributing information to that outcome.

Summary assessment of risk of bias

To draw conclusions about the overall risk of bias within or across trials it is necessary to summarise assessments across items in the tool for each outcome within each

trial. In doing this, review authors must decide which domains are most important in the context of the review, ideally when writing their protocol. For example, for highly subjective outcomes such as pain, blinding of participants is critical. The way that summary judgments of risk of bias are reached should be explicit and should be informed by empirical evidence of bias when it exists, likely direction of bias, and likely magnitude of bias. Table 3 provides a suggested framework for making summary assessments of the risk of bias for important outcomes within and across trials.

Assessments of risk of bias and synthesis of results

Summary assessments of the risk of bias for an outcome within each trial should inform the meta-analysis. The two preferable analytical strategies are to restrict the primary meta-analysis to studies at low risk of bias or to present meta-analyses stratified according to risk of bias. The choice between these strategies should be based on the context of the particular review and the balance between the potential for bias and the loss of precision when studies at high or unclear risk of bias are excluded. Meta-regression can be used to compare results from studies at high and low risk of bias, but such comparisons lack power,[15] and lack of a significant difference should not be interpreted as implying the absence of bias.

A third strategy is to present a meta-analysis of all studies while providing a summary of the risk of bias across studies. However, this runs the risk that bias is downplayed in the discussion and conclusions of a review, so that decisions continue to be based, at least in part, on flawed evidence. This risk could be reduced by incorporating summary assessments into broader, but explicit, measures of the quality of evidence for each important outcome, for example using the GRADE system.[16] This can help to ensure that judgments about the risk of bias, as well as other factors affecting the quality of evidence (such as imprecision, heterogeneity, and publication bias), are considered when interpreting the results of systematic reviews.[17] [18]

Discussion

Discrepancies between the results of different systematic reviews examining the same question[19] [20] and between meta-analyses and subsequent large trials[21] have shown that the results of meta-analyses can be biased, which may be partly caused by biased results in the trials they include. We believe our risk of bias tool is one of the most comprehensive approaches to assessing the potential for bias in randomised trials included in systematic reviews or meta-analyses. Inclusion of details of trial conduct, on which judgments of risk of bias are based, provides greater transparency than previous approaches, allowing readers to decide whether they agree with the judgments made. There is continuing uncertainty, and great variation in practice, over how to assess potential for bias in specific domains within trials, how to summarise bias assessments across such domains, and how to incorporate bias assessments into meta-analyses.

A recent study has found that the tool takes longer to complete than other tools (the investigators took a mean of 8.8 minutes per person for a single predetermined outcome using our tool compared with 1.5 minutes for a previous rating scale for quality of reporting).[22] The reliability of the tool has not been extensively studied, although the same authors observed that larger effect sizes were observed on

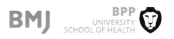

average in studies rated as at high risk of bias compared with studies at low risk of bias.[22]

By explicitly incorporating judgments into the tool, we acknowledge that agreements between assessors may not be as high as for some other tools. However, we also explicitly target the risk of bias rather than reported characteristics of the trial. It would be easier to assess whether a drop-out rate exceeds 20% than whether a drop-out rate of 21% introduces an important risk of bias, but there is no guarantee that results from a study with a drop-out rate lower than 20% are at low risk of bias. Preliminary evidence suggests that incomplete outcome data and selective reporting are the most difficult items to assess; kappa measures of agreement of 0.32 (fair) and 0.13 (slight) respectively have been reported for these.[22] It is important that guidance and training materials continue to be developed for all aspects of the tool, but particularly these two.

We hope that widespread adoption and implementation of the risk of bias tool, both within and outside the Cochrane Collaboration, will facilitate improved appraisal of evidence by healthcare decision makers and patients and ultimately lead to better healthcare. Improved understanding of the ways in which flaws in trial conduct may bias their results should also lead to better trials and more reliable evidence. Risk of bias assessments should continue to evolve, taking into account any new empirical evidence and the practical experience of authors of systematic reviews.

Contributors: All authors contributed to the drafting and editing of the manuscript. JPTH, DGA, PCG, PJ, DM, ADO, KFS and JACS contributed to the chapter in the *Cochrane Handbook for Systematic Reviews of Interventions* on which the paper is based. JPTH will act as guarantor.

Development meeting participants (May 2005): Doug Altman (co-lead), Gerd Antes, Chris Cates, Jon Deeks, Peter Gøtzsche, Julian Higgins (co-lead), Sally Hopewell, Peter Jüni (organising committee), Steff Lewis, Philippa Middleton, David Moher (organising committee), Andy Oxman, Ken Schulz (organising committee), Nandi Siegfried, Jonathan Sterne, Simon Thompson.

Other contributors to tool development: Hilda Bastian, Rachelle Buchbinder, Iain Chalmers, Miranda Cumpston, Sally Green, Peter Herbison, Victor Montori, Hannah Rothstein, Georgia Salanti, Guido Schwarzer, Ian Shrier, Jayne Tierney, Ian White and Paula Williamson.

Evaluation meeting participants (March 2010): Doug Altman (organising committee), Elaine Beller, Sally Bell-Syer, Chris Cates, Rachel Churchill, June Cody, Jonathan Cook, Christian Gluud, Julian Higgins (organising committee), Sally Hopewell, Hayley Jones, Peter Jüni, Monica Kjeldstrøm, Toby Lasserson, Allyson Lipp, Lara Maxwell, Joanne McKenzie, Craig Ramsey, Barney Reeves, Jelena Savović (co-lead), Jonathan Sterne (co-lead), David Tovey, Laura Weeks (organising committee).

Other contributors to tool evaluation: Isabelle Boutron, David Moher (organising committee), Lucy Turner.

Funding: The development and evaluation of the risk of bias tool was funded in part by The Cochrane Collaboration. The views expressed in this article are those of the authors and not necessarily those of The Cochrane Collaboration or its registered entities, committees or working groups.. JPTH was also funded by MRC grant number U.1052.00.011. DGA was funded by Cancer Research UK grant number C-5592. DM was funded by a University Research Chair (University of Ottawa). The Canadian Institutes of Health Research provides financial support to the Cochrane Bias Methods Group.

Competing interests: All authors have completed the ICJME unified disclosure form at www.icmje.org/coi_disclosure.pdf (available on request from the corresponding author) and declare support from the Cochrane Collaboration for the development and evaluation of the tool described; they have no financial relationships with any organisations that might have an interest in the submitted work in the previous three years and no other relationships or activities that could appear to have influenced the submitted work.

Provenance and peer review: Not commissioned; externally peer reviewed.

1   Kleijnen J, Gøtzsche P, Kunz RH, Oxman AD, Chalmers I. So what's so special about randomisation? In: Maynard A, Chalmers I, eds. *Non-random reflections on health services research: on the 25th anniversary of Archie Cochrane's Effectiveness and Efficiency* . BMJ Books, 1997:93-106.
2   Wood L, Egger M, Gluud LL, Schulz K, Jüni P, Altman DG, et al. Empirical evidence of bias in treatment effect estimates in controlled trials with different interventions and outcomes: meta-epidemiological study. *BMJ* 2008;336:601-5.
3   Egger M, Davey Smith G, Altman DG, eds. *Systematic reviews in health care: meta-analysis in context* . BMJ Books, 2001.
4   Moher D, Jadad AR, Nichol G, Penman M, Tugwell P, Walsh S. Assessing the quality of randomized controlled trials—an annotated bibliography of scales and checklists. *Controlled Clin Trials* 1995;12:62-73.
5   Jüni P, Altman DG, Egger M. Systematic reviews in health care: assessing the quality of controlled clinical trials. *BMJ* 2001;323:42-6.
6   West S, King V, Carey TS, Lohr KN, McKoy N, Sutton SF, et al. *Systems to rate the strength of scientific evidence. Evidence report/technology assessment no 47.* AHRQ publication No 02-E016. Agency for Healthcare Research and Quality, 2002.
7   Crowe M, Sheppard L. A review of critical appraisal tools show they lack rigor: alternative tool structure is proposed. *J Clin Epidemiol* 2011;64:79-89.
8   Lundh A, Gøtzsche PC. Recommendations by Cochrane Review Groups for assessment of the risk of bias in studies. *BMC Med Res Methodol* 2008;8:22.
9   Higgins JPT, Green S, eds. *Cochrane handbook for systematic reviews of interventions* . Wiley, 2008.
10 Greenland S, O'Rourke K. On the bias produced by quality scores in meta-analysis, and a hierarchical view of proposed solutions. *Biostatistics* 2001;2:463-71.
11 Jüni P, Witschi A, Bloch R, Egger M. The hazards of scoring the quality of clinical trials for meta-analysis. *JAMA* 1999;282:1054-60.
12 Gluud LL. Bias in clinical intervention research. *Am J Epidemiol* 2006;163:493-501.
13 Higgins JPT, Altman DG. Assessing risk of bias in included studies. In: Higgins JPT, Green S, eds. *Cochrane handbook for systematic reviews of interventions* . Wiley, 2008:187-241.
14 Kredo T, Van der Walt J-S, Siegfried N, Cohen K. Therapeutic drug monitoring of antiretrovirals for people with HIV. *Cochrane Database Syst Rev* 2009;3:CD007268.
15 Higgins JPT, Thompson SG. Controlling the risk of spurious findings from meta-regression. *Stat Med* 2004;23:1663-82.
16 Guyatt GH, Oxman AD, Vist GE, Zunz R, Falck-Ytter Y, Alonso-Coello P, et al. GRADE: an emerging consensus on rating quality of evidence and strength of recommendations. *BMJ* 2008;336:924-6.
17 Schünemann HJ, Oxman AD, Higgins JPT, Vist GE, Glasziou P, Guyatt GH, et al. Presenting results and "Summary of findings" tables. In: Higgins JPT, Green S, eds. *Cochrane handbook for systematic reviews of interventions* . Wiley, 2008:335-8.
18 Schünemann HJ, Oxman AD, Vist GE, Higgins JPT, Deeks JJ, Glasziou P, et al. Interpreting results and drawing conclusions. In: Higgins JPT, Green S, eds. *Cochrane handbook for systematic reviews of interventions* . Wiley, 2008:359-87.
19 Leizorovicz A, Haugh MC, Chapuis FR, Samama MM, Boissel JP. Low molecular weight heparin in prevention of perioperative thrombosis. *BMJ* 1992;305:913-20.
20 Nurmohamed MT, Rosendaal FR, Buller HR, Dekker E, Hommes DW, Vandenbroucke JP, et al. Low-molecular-weight heparin versus standard heparin in general and orthopaedic surgery: a meta-analysis. *Lancet* 1992;340:152-6.
21 Lelorier J, Benhaddad A, Lapierre J, Derderian F. Discrepancies between meta-analyses and subsequent large randomized, controlled trials. *N Engl J Med* 1997;337:536-42.
22 Hartling L, Ospina M, Liang Y, Dryden DM, Hooton N, Krebs SJ, et al. Risk of bias versus quality assessment of randomised controlled trials: cross sectional study. *BMJ* 2009;339:b4012.

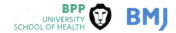

Taking healthcare interventions from trial to practice

Paul Glasziou, professor[1], Iain Chalmers, coordinator (James Lind Initiative)[2], Douglas G Altman, professor of statistics in medicine[3], Hilda Bastian, editor in chief[4], Isabelle Boutron, statistician[5], Anne Brice, information specialist[1], Gro Jamtvedt, executive director[6], Andrew Farmer, professor of general practice[1], Davina Ghersi, team leader[7], Trish Groves, deputy editor[8], Carl Heneghan, director, Cen[t] for Evidence Based Medicine[1], Sophie Hill, researcher[9], Simon Lewin, researcher[6], Susan Michie, professor of health psychology[10], Rafael Perera, researcher[1], Valerie Pomeroy, professor of neurorehabilitation[11], Julie Tilson, assistant professor[12], Sasha Shepperd, researcher[1], John W Williams, professor of medicine and psychiatry[13]

[1]Department of Public Health and Primary Care, University of Oxford, Oxford OX3 7LF

[2]James Lind Initiative, Oxford OX2 7LG

[3]Centre for Statistics in Medicine, Oxford OX2 6UD

[4]German Institute for Quality and Efficiency in Health Care, Cologne, Germany

[5]INSERM, Université Paris, Paris, France

[6]Norwegian Knowledge Centre for the Health Services, Oslo, Norway

[7]Department of Research Policy and Cooperation, World Health Organization, Geneva

[8]BMJ, London

[9]Centre for Health Communication and Participation, Australian Institute for Primary Care, La Trobe University, Victoria, Australia

[10]Division of Psychology and Language Sciences, University College London, London WC1E 7HB

[11]Health and Social Sciences Research Institute, Faculty of Health, University of East Anglia, Norwich

[12]Division of Biokinesiology and Physical Therapy, University of Southern California, Los Angeles, CA, USA

[13]Duke Evidence-based Practice Center, Duke University and Durham VA Medical Center Durham, NC, USA

Correspondence to: P Glasziou paul.glasziou@dphpc.ox.ac.uk

Cite this as: *BMJ* 2010;341:c3852

DOI: 10.1136/bmj.c3852

http://www.bmj.com/content/341/bmj.c3852

Much healthcare research is currently wasted because its findings are unusable.[1] Published reports of intervention trials often focus on the results and fail to describe interventions adequately. For example, a review of 80 studies selected for the journal *Evidence Based Medicine* as both valid and important for clinical practice found that clinicians could replicate the intervention in only half the studies.[2] Interventions may be used incorrectly or not at all if there is inadequate detail in the trial protocol, on the conduct of the trial, in systematic reviews and guidelines, and finally during implementation (fig 1). This is an unnecessary but remediable waste, as we discuss below.

Study protocol

The methods section in a protocol should provide a description of the intervention(s) (whether active, usual practice, or placebo) that is sufficiently detailed to enable people with appropriate expertise to reproduce them. This should include:

- What were the "contents," including all constituent components, materials, and resources and their quality
- Who delivered the intervention, including their expertise, additional training, and support
- Where the intervention was delivered (the setting)
- How and when the intervention was delivered: the dose, the schedule (intensity, frequency, duration), and interaction
- The degree of flexibility permissible, including options and decision points.[3]

This list is readily adaptable for interventions beyond clinical treatments and encounters—for example, to health systems and other complex interventions. Attention should be paid to the different meanings that terms such as counselling or physical therapy may have in different settings.

Space constraints in trial registration databases and scientific journals may restrict full reporting of interventions. Potential solutions include complying with WHO requirements for reporting interventions, adding web hyperlinks to trial registration records and other documentation,[4] as recommended by signatories to the Ottawa statement (ottawagroup.ohri.ca) and on other websites where protocols are reported.

ABSTRACT

The results of thousands of trials are never acted on because their published reports do not describe the interventions in enough detail. How can we improve the reporting?

The development and description of treatment sched[ule] may take considerable planning, particularly for n[on] drug interventions. Figure 2 shows the development [of] conventional physical therapy interventions as a precu[rsor] to studies evaluating novel interventions for reco[very] of movement after stroke.[5] Semistructured intervi[ew] and focus groups were used to capture the content [of] conventional physical therapy interventions.[5]

Study fidelity: planned versus actual treatment

Trial reports should describe the extent to which [the] intervention, as delivered, was consistent with the proto[col]. Fidelity can have several dimensions: whether compone[nts] are delivered as prescribed (adherence); the amount [of] exposure to the content; the extent to which the deliv[ery] was aligned with the underpinning theory (quality); [the] degree to which participants engaged in[6] or modified [the] intervention. Poor fidelity will lead to unclear or mislead[ing] conclusions.

Despite its importance, fidelity of the intervention [is] often not reported: only 25 of 80 (31%) prevention stud[ies] reported evidence of fidelity,[6] and only 69 of 192 (3[6%]) drug studies documented assessment of adherence [to] treatment—the simplest measure of fidelity.[7]

Assessment of fidelity may require qualitative a[nd] quantitative methods. For example, a trial compar[ing] the effect of two diagnostic tests for malaria delive[red] inconclusive results, but a parallel qualitative study show[ed] that in areas of high malaria prevalence clinicians trea[t] malaria regardless of the random allocation.[8] Likewise, a large trial of an intervention to increase physical activ[ity] in sedentary adults, coding of session audiotapes show[ed] that only 42% of intervention techniques were delivered [as] specified in the protocol.[9]

Interventions can involve several actors. Though clinicia[ns] may deliver the intervention, participants may not adh[ere] to it. Hence the role of both clinician and participant nee[d]

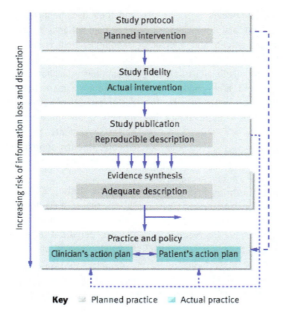

Fig 1 Distortion or loss of information about the true intervention can occur at each of four stages and the intervention may not reach practice without good reporting and trial fidelity (shaded boxes)

to be described. An example of good practice is the DiGEM trial of self monitoring of blood glucose concentrations,[10] for which the nurse training manual describes the intervention and timing of delivery in detail, with the intended effect and the required level of knowledge, skills, and behaviour for the research nurse and the person with diabetes.

Measures to improve and assess fidelity at the trial protocol stage include:

- Designing the intervention using a recognised theoretical framework

- Producing a manual or written instructions for the interventions

- Training all study members responsible for protocol delivery

- Observing delivery

- Using checklists to ensure competency and standardisation of delivery

- Providing support material for trial participants that promotes adherence.

Any drift away from fidelity during the trial should be reported when the study is published.

Publication of single studies

The Uniform Requirements for Manuscripts Submitted to Biomedical Journals have for many years advised authors to "Describe statistical methods with enough detail to enable

a knowledgeable reader with access to the original data to verify the reported results." (www.icmje.org)

It is unclear why this suggestion has not been extended to all aspects of the research methods. The need to provide detailed information about interventions has been recognised in several guidelines for reporting research, the best known of which is the CONSORT (Consolidated Standards of Reporting Trials) statement.[11] And the 2010 update of the CONSORT statement requires authors to describe "the interventions for each group with sufficient details to allow replication, including how and when they were actually administered."

Despite the CONSORT guidelines and advice on good reporting of interventions, reporting is currently poor (table). For example, only 13% of papers on back pain reported reproducible interventions.[12] A review of 158 reports of randomised controlled trials in surgery showed that important components of the intervention (such as anaesthesia protocol or perioperative management) were reported in less than half.[13] Furthermore, only 41% reported the intervention actually administered as opposed to the intervention intended in the protocol.[13]

Since 2001, extensions to CONSORT have focused on specific types of intervention with detailed recommendations on reporting interventions. For example, the extension to trials of non-drug treatments[15] recommended the reporting of precise details of both the experimental treatment and comparator, including a description of the different components of the interventions and, when applicable, descriptions of the procedure for tailoring the interventions to individual participants; details of how the interventions were standardised, and details of how adherence to the protocol of care providers was assessed or enhanced. The extensions for other types of study have not directly tackled ability to replicate interventions, although the WIDER (Workgroup for Intervention Development and Evaluation Research) group of journal editors has given recommendations to ensure behavioural interventions can be replicated.[16]

Adequate reporting is difficult and needs greater attention from authors, peer reviewers, and journals. Trials of complex interventions particularly may benefit from innovative communication methods such as graphic techniques,[17] video, and audio. For example, videos are available to guide use of the WHO safe surgery checklist.[18]

Table 1 Summary of studies that assessed whether interventions in published trial reports could be replicated

Clinical area	No of Trials	No (%) replicable	Methods of assessment
Back pain[12]	24	3 (13)	Information sufficient for consumers
Surgical procedures[13]	158	138 (87)	Required only that "some" detail was provided, not sufficient for replication; 41% also provided some detail on actual surgery used
Weight loss interventions[14]	63	62 (98)	Compliance with item 4 of CONSORT statement*
Range of topics published in *Evidence Based Medicine*[2]	55	36 (65)	Two general practitioners were independently asked whether they could use this treatment with patients if they saw them tomorrow

*2001 update.[11]

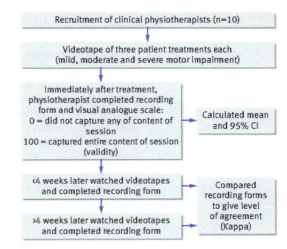

Fig 2 Illustration of methods to develop a physical therapy treatment schedule[5]

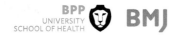

Synthesis of evidence and systematic reviews

Interventions will usually vary across trials in a systematic review, reflecting differing inclusion criteria and specific aspects of the intervention. Even for relatively simple interventions, such as antibiotics for acute sinusitis, the specific antibiotic, dose, duration, and timing may vary. For more complex interventions, such as strategies to implement clinical practice guidelines, heterogeneity is greater.[19]

For the review user a central question is: "Which intervention should we use when there are multiple versions in a review?" For example, a review reported that exercise for patients with osteoarthritis of the knee can reduce pain and improve function.[20] However, almost all studies in the review used different types and doses of exercise. If a review shows a collective intervention to be effective, the user is challenged to determine which configuration, elements, or dose of the intervention should be implemented for their patients or setting. Methods to guide this are poorly developed. (Note: identical problems occur in guideline development.)

During synthesis of evidence, the intervention description may be modified at several stages:

The review protocol—An intervention may be inadequately conceptualised at the protocol stage

Conducting the review—Authors may not consider the features of an intervention that could affect implementation and instead focus on classifying interventions for exploring heterogeneity

Dissemination—When the review enters the media, the description of the intervention may be altered

This complicates decisions about which configuration of the intervention to implement.

With rare exceptions[21] reviewers seldom attempt to improve descriptions of interventions. Conceptual frameworks may facilitate the classification and description of interventions. For example, a review of "audit and feedback" classified interventions according to intensity and provided examples to illustrate different intensities.[22] This categorisation was intuitive and not based on theory. Using theory may lead to conceptually more coherent categories and therefore more meaningful results.

Mapping the components of an intervention

Specifying the components within interventions in a review can help identify similarities and differences, allowing the effective "ingredients" to be defined. For example, Rubenstein used cross-case qualitative analysis to assess whether specific design features of collaborative care interventions were associated with greater effect on depression compared with usual care.[23] This qualitative analysis looked closely at features that occurred in studies with greater effects, generating hypotheses about the most important components of the intervention. Core components may also be identified by surveying trialists. For example, Langhorne et al used all trials of "stroke units" to identify key components then surveyed the trialists' collaboration to find out which components they had used and derive a composite intervention.[21]

Taxonomies

One method of identifying the active ingredient(s) of an intervention is to systematically specify them—and control comparison conditions—using standardised taxonomies

and then use meta-regression to show effects hidden more conventional methods of synthesising evidence.[24] Taxonomies help ensure a planned approach to analys particularly when heterogeneity prevents meta-analys Taxonomies facilitate the process of accumulati knowledge across heterogeneous studies, making easier to update reviews and identify gaps. Mechanis underlying an intervention can be investigated by linki active ingredients to hypothesised causal mechanisr (theory) through approaches such as "realist synthesis" consensus among content experts.

Using the study

Unless there is clarity about what interventions involv patients and health professionals cannot ensure th receive beneficial interventions or avoid unhelpful harmful interventions.

Patients, practitioners, and policy makers learn abc interventions directly from trials and systematic reviev or, more commonly, from intermediaries and seconda sources (websites, advice centres, media, clinical practi guidelines, librarians) or practitioners. The details evaluated interventions should be readily available in t public domain. The minimal elements of knowledge th patients (or the providers of information to patients) ne about the intervention are who, what, when, and ho as we set out above. Additionally, clinicians may ne information about skills, equipment, or referral sources provide effective treatment. The box gives our proposals increase the usefulness of research reports (box).

> ### ACTIONS TO IMPROVE USEFULNESS OF RESEARCH REPORTS
>
> - When planning trials, researchers should work with end users to develop and deliver the interventions. Clear specifications of the components of the intervention should be planned and reported
> - Researchers and funders should improve the description of interventions (including "usual practice") in protocols and pay attention to the fidelity of an intervention
> - A stable "intervention bank" should be established (eg, videos, manuals, and fidelity tools linked to trial registratior number) to overcome the problem of word restrictions in journals, etc
> - Systematic reviews should include a summary table describing study interventions, with links to trial publications and other resources relevant to replicating the interventions
> - The reporting standards for interventions in trials (CONSORT, etc) and systematic reviews (PRISMA[26]) should be improved and standardised (specific checklists)

We thank Mike Clarke and the reviewers for helpful comments and Mary Hodgkinson for organising meetings. The costs of the meeting were in part covered by PG's NIHR fellowship.

Contributors and sources: PG organised and IC chaired a two day consensus meeting of the authors to discuss the problems of reporting trial interventions, develop a guide on describing interventions throughout the research process, and prioritise recommendations to reduce information distortion and loss. All authors contributed to discussions and writing of the paper.

Competing interests: All authors have completed the unified competing interest form at www.icmje.org/coi_disclosure.pdf (available on request from the corresponding author) and declare no support from any organisation for the submitted work and no financial relationships with any organisation that might have an interest in the submitted work in the previous three years; TG is an editor at the *BMJ* but was not involved in the peer review process. is an employee of the World Health Organization and works on trial registration. DA is an executive member of the EQUATOR network.

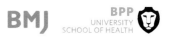

Provenance and peer review: Not commissioned; externally peer reviewed.

1   Chalmers I, Glasziou P. Avoidable waste in the production and reporting of research evidence. *Lancet* 2009;374:86-9.

2   Glasziou P, Meats E, Heneghan C, Shepperd S. What is missing from descriptions of treatment in trials and reviews? *BMJ* 2008;336:1472-4.

3   Lustria ML, Cortese J, Noar SM, Glueckauf RL. Computer tailored health interventions delivered over the web: review and analysis of key components. *Patient Educ Counsel* 2009;74:156-73.

4   Chan A-W. Bias, spin, and misreporting: time for full access to trial protocols and results. *PLoS Med* 2008;5:e230.

5   Pomeroy VM, Cooke E, Hamilton S, Whittet A, Tallis RC. Development of a schedule of current physiotherapy treatment used to improve movement control and functional use of the lower limb after stroke: a precursor to a clinical trial. *Neurorehabil Neural Repair* 2005;19:350-9.

6   Dane AV, Schneider BH. Program integrity in primary and early secondary prevention: are implementation effects out of control? *Clin Psychol Rev* 1998;18:23-45.

7   Gossec L, Tubach F, Dougados M, Ravaud P. Reporting of adherence to medication in recent randomized controlled trials of 6 chronic diseases: a systematic literature review. *Am J Med Sci* 2007;334:248-54.

8   Lubell Y, Reyburn H, Mbakilwa H, Mwangi R, Chonya S, Whitty CJ, et al. The impact of response to the results of diagnostic tests for malaria: cost-benefit analysis. *BMJ* 2008;336:202-5.

9   Hardeman W, Michie S, Fanshawe T, Prevost AT, McLoughlin K, Kinmonth AL. Fidelity of delivery of a physical activity intervention: Predictors and consequences. *Psychol Health* 2008;23:11-24.

10   Farmer A, Wade A, French D, Simon J, Yudkin P, Gray A, et al. Blood glucose self-monitoring in type 2 diabetes: a randomised controlled trial. *Health Technol Assess* 2009;13:1-72.

11   Moher D, Schulz KF, Altman DG. The CONSORT statement: revised recommendations for improving the quality of reports of parallel-group randomized trials. *Ann Intern Med* 2001;134:657-62.

12   Glenton C, Underland V, Kho M, Pennick V, Oxman AD. Summaries of findings, descriptions of treatments, and information about adverse effects would make reviews more informative. *J Clin Epidemiol* 2006;59:770-8.

13   Jacquier I, Boutron I, Moher D, Roy C, Ravaud P. The reporting of randomized clinical trials using a surgical intervention is in need of immediate improvement: a systematic review. *Ann Surg* 2006;244:677-83.

14   Thabane L, Chu R, Cuddy K, Douketis J. What is the quality of reporting in weight loss intervention studies? A systematic review of randomized controlled trials. *Int J Obes (Lond)* 2007.

15   Boutron I, Moher D, Altman DG, Schulz K, Ravaud P, for the CONSORT group. Methods and processes of the CONSORT group: example of an extension for trials assessing nonpharmacologic treatments. *Ann Intern Med* 2008:W60-W67.

16   Workgroup for Intervention Development and Evaluation Research. WIDER recommendations to improve reporting of the content of behaviour change interventions. 2009. http://interventiondesign.co.uk/wp-content/uploads/2009/02/wider-recommendations.pdf.

17   Perera R, Heneghan C, Yudkin P. Graphical method for depicting randomised trials of complex interventions. *BMJ* 2007;334:127-9.

18   WHO Safe Surgery Checklist. Instructional videos. www.who.int/patientsafety/safesurgery/tools_resources/en/index.html.

19   Craig P, Dieppe P, Macintyre S, Michie S, Nazareth I, et al. Developing and evaluating complex interventions: the new Medical Research Council guidance. *BMJ* 2008;337:a1655.

20   Fransen M, McConnell S. Exercise for osteoarthritis of the knee. *Cochrane Database Syst Rev* 2008;4:CD004376.

21   Langhorne P, Pollock A, with the Stroke Unit Trialists Collaboration. What are the components of effective stroke unit care? *Age Ageing* 2002;31:365-71.

22   Jamtvedt G, Young JM, Kristoffersen DT, O'Brien MA, Oxman AD. Audit and feedback: effects on professional practice and health care outcomes. *Cochrane Database Syst Rev* 2006;2:CD000259.

23   Rubenstein LV, Williams Jr JW, Danz M, Shekelle P. Evidence synthesis for determining the key features of effective depression interventions. 2009. www.hsrd.research.va.gov/publications/esp/#depression.

24   Abraham C, Michie S. A taxonomy of behavior change techniques used in interventions. *Health Psychol* 2008;27:379-87.

25   Michie S, Abraham C. Advancing the science of behaviour change: a plea for scientific reporting. *Addiction* 2008;103:1409-10.

26   Liberati A, Altman DG, Tetzlaff J, Mulrow C, Gøtzsche PC, Ioannidis JP, et al. The PRISMA statement for reporting systematic reviews and meta-analyses of studies that evaluate healthcare interventions: explanation and elaboration. *BMJ* 2009;339:b2700.

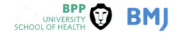

Clinical prediction rules

Simon T Adams, clinical research fellow[1], Stephen H Leveson, professor of surgery[2]

[1]York Hospital, York YO31 8HE, UK

[2]Hull-York Medical School, Learning and Research Centre, York Hospital

Correspondence to: S Adams rpbgt@hotmail.com

Cite this as: *BMJ* 2012;344:d8312

DOI: 10.1136/bmj.d8312

http://www.bmj.com/content/344/bmj.d8312

In many ways much of the art of medicine boils down to playing the percentages and predicting outcomes. For example, when clinicians take a history from a patient they ask the questions that they think are the most likely to provide them with the information they need to make a diagnosis. They might then order the tests that they think are the most likely to support or refute their various differential diagnoses. With each new piece of the puzzle some hypotheses will become more likely and others less likely. At the end of the process the clinician will decide which treatment is likely to result in the most favourable outcome for the patient, based on the information they have obtained.

Given that the above process is the underlying principle of clinical practice, and bearing in mind the ever increasing time constraints imposed on people, it is unsurprising that a great deal of work has been done to help clinicians and patients make decisions. This work is referred to by many names: prediction rules, probability assessments, prediction models, decision rules, risk scores, etc. All describe the combination of multiple predictors, such as patient characteristics and investigation results, to estimate the probability of a certain outcome or to identify which intervention is most likely to be effective.[1] [2] Predictors are identified by "data mining"—the process of selecting, exploring, and modelling large amounts of data in order to discover unknown patterns or relations.[3]

Ideally, a reliable predictive factor or model would combine both a high sensitivity with a high specificity.[4] [5] In other words it would correctly identify as high a proportion as possible of the patients fated to have the outcome in question (sensitivity) while excluding those who will not have the outcome (specificity).[6] In the table sensitivity can be defined as A÷(A+C) and specificity as D÷(B+D).

A good predictive factor is not the same as a strong risk factor.[4] The positive predictive value of a predictive factor or model refers to its accuracy in terms of the proportion of patients correctly predicted to have the outcome in question (A÷(A+B) in the table).[7] A risk factor can be identified by calculating the relative risk (or odds ratio) of an outcome in patients with the factor in question compared with patients without it.[4] If, however, the factor identified or the outcome being used is uncommon, it is of little clinical use as a predictive factor.[4] [7]

A good predictive factor or model shows a good fit between the probabilities calculated from the model and the outcomes actually observed, while also accurately discriminating between patients with and without the outcome.[4] [5] For example, if all patients with a measured observation of ≥0.5 die and all patients with the measured observation <0.5 survive then the observed factor is a perfect predictor of survival.

Unfortunately, as a general rule sensitivity and specificity are mutually exclusive—as one rises the other falls. Since both are important to the development of predictive models receiver-operating characteristic (ROC) curves are used to visualise the trade-off between the two and express the overall accuracy of the model (fig 1).[4] [8] [9] Sensitivity (true

ABSTRACT

Clinical prediction rules are mathematical tools that are intended to guide clinicians in their everyday decision making. The popularity of such rules has increased greatly over the past few years. This article outlines the concepts underlying their development and the pros and cons of their use

positive) is plotted on the y axis and 1–specificity (false positive) is plotted on the x axis.[4] [9] The closer a point to the top left of the graph then the higher the area under the curve and the more accurate or useful a predictive factor can be said to be.[4] [8] [9] Conversely a plot in the degree diagonal (denoting an area under the curve of 50%) indicates a test no more accurate than chance.[4] [8] [9] Where the limits of acceptability are set is arbitrary and depends on several factors such as the severity of the outcome and the potential negative consequences of the test.[4] [9]

Establishing a clinical prediction rule

The establishment of a prediction model in clinical practice requires four distinct phases:

Development—Identification of predictors from an observational study

Validation—Testing of the rule in a separate population to see if it remains reliable

Impact analysis—Measurement of the usefulness of the rule in the clinical setting in terms of cost-benefit, patient satisfaction, time/resource allocation, etc

Implementation—Widespread acceptance and adoption of the rule in clinical practice.

For a prediction rule to gain popularity each of the first three steps needs to be satisfactorily completed before the fourth stage.[1] Validation in a suitably powered cohort study or controlled trial is particularly important because there is no guarantee that a predictor will be accurate outside the original data set.[1] [2] Indeed validation usually shows a reduction in accuracy compared to that in the original study.[1] [10] [11] [12] Reliability is essentially the reproducibility of measurement—that is, if the same test were applied under the same circumstances how similar the results would be.

Despite the long running controversy concerning the usefulness and application the popularity of clinical prediction rules has been shown to be greater now than ever.[1] [13] [14] A Medline search by Toll and colleagues in 2008 showed that the number of papers discussing prediction rules has more than doubled in recent years (6744 papers in 1995 versus 15 662 in 2005).[1] Most publications, however, concern the development of new rules, with few articles describing validation and almost none confirming their clinical impact.[1] There are several possible reasons why validation and impact analysis are so often overlooked. Perhaps the most important are that neither validity nor reliability can be exactly quantified and that establishing validity requires investigators to consider several different aspects (face validity, content validity, construct validity, criterion validity, etc).[15] [16]

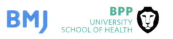

Table 1 Tabular representation of predicted versus actual outcomes of a predictive model

	Actual outcome	
Predicted outcome	**Positive**	**Negative**
Positive	A (true positive)	B (false positive)
Negative	C (false negative)	D (true negative)

Advantages and disadvantages of prediction rules

When appropriately developed and validated, prediction models have inherent advantages over human clinical decision making. Firstly, the statistical models can accommodate many more factors than the human brain is capable of taking into consideration.[17] Secondly, if given identical data a statistical model will always give the same result whereas human clinical judgment has been shown to result in both inconsistency and disparity, especially with less experienced clinicians.[17] [18] Finally, and perhaps most importantly, several prediction models have been shown to be more accurate than clinical judgment alone.[14] [17] [18] [19] [20] [21] So why are such models not used more readily in every practice?

Liao and Mark proposed in 2003 that resistance to adopting prediction models may reflect tacit acknowledgment that clinicians do not know how to take advantage of such tools.[17] They also suggested that such tools may not be thought user friendly and may not take into account the continual, dynamic way in which humans gather clinical information.[17] Their final reason for low implementation of clinical prediction rules is the sheer number of models available.[17] If multiple prediction rules exist for the same problem identifying the best one is difficult. Not only is it potentially very time consuming but differences in the methods used in the studies on which they are based may make reliable comparison impossible.[11] [22] Part of the reason for the large number of prediction rules may be the wide variety of ways in which such tools can be developed.

Types of prediction model

In 2006 Grobman and Stamilio described five main methods used to develop clinical prediction models: scoring systems derived from univariate analysis, prediction models based on multivariate analysis, nomograms, artificial neural networks, and decision trees.

Scoring systems derived from univariate analysis

Factors shown to be significantly related to the outcome in observational studies are allocated a score or "weight." The cumulative final score of all the risk factors present in a patient is used as an indicator of the likelihood of the outcome occurring.[4] Well known examples of this type of prediction model include the Alvarado score for acute appendicitis and the modified Glasgow score for acute pancreatitis.[23] [24] These models are simple to devise and use but their accuracy is affected by the potential inclusion of non-independent risk factors and the arbitrary manner in which factors are weighted.[4]

Prediction models based on multivariate analysis

These are developed in a similar manner to the above scoring systems except that the analysis of the results from the observational study is more refined and therefore less likely to include any non-independent factors. The models typically use logistic regression analysis, which has the added advantage of expressing the relation between the predictive factors and the outcome in the form of odds ratios (the probability of an outcome occurring versus the probability that it will not).[4] These are relatively easy to interpret and can also be used to assign weights in a less arbitrary fashion than in univariate models.[4] [25] Nevertheless, multivariate analysis techniques are not completely reliable in eliminating bias from interaction of independent variables.[4] Models using logistic regression are often well suited to being represented as a nomogram (see below).[3]

Nomograms

Nomograms are graphical calculating devices that represent mathematical relations or laws and allow the user to rapidly calculate complicated formulas to a practical precision (fig 2).[26] Nomograms may be as simple as the markings on a thermometer or more complex, such as the Siggaard-Andersen chart used to diagnose acid-base blood disorders.[27] The mathematics and statistics used to develop a nomogram can be equally simplistic or intricate.[4] The advantage of nomograms is that the final prediction tool created is generally comparatively simple to use and in some cases more accurate than other prediction models for the same clinical problem.[4] [28] Other nomograms in common clinical use include those used to predict the likelihood of a patient having prostate cancer from their clinical examination and prostate specific antigen levels and those used to predict the peak expiratory flow rate of asthmatic patients based on their age and height.[29] [30]

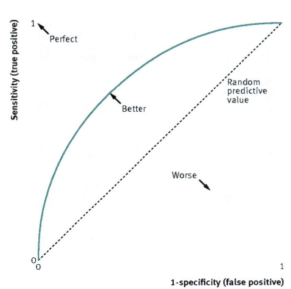

Fig 1 Receiver-operating characteristic (ROC) curve

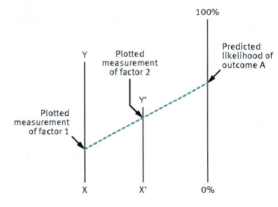

Fig 2 Simplified representation of a basic nomogram

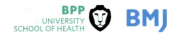

Prediction using artificial neural networks

Artificial neural networks are mathematical or computational models based on the operation of biological neural networks.[31] In biology, a nerve cell (or neuron) will receive input from numerous other nerve cells. It will then process all of the input it receives and either send off an action potential or not. Because these nerve cells are all interconnected they are referred to as networks. Artificial neural networks function along similar lines: multiple sources of information (input) are fed into the software program, which interprets it and produces a dichotomous output (fig 3). The main advantage of neural networks is that they can "learn" mathematical relations between a series of input variables and the corresponding output.[32] [33] [34] [35] This is achieved by inputting a set of data containing both the input data (the predictor variables) as well as the outcomes.[32] [33] With each new data set entered the neural network is able to adjust the internal weights of the various pieces of input data and calculate the probability of a specific outcome.[32]

Neural networks require little formal statistical training to develop and can implicitly detect complex non-linear relations between independent and dependent variables as well as all possible interactions between predictor variables.[32] [33] However, they have a limited ability to explicitly identify possible causal relations, they are hard to use at the bedside, and they require greater computational resources than other prediction models.[32] [33] They are also prone to "overfitting"—when too many data sets are used in training the network causing it to effectively memorise the noise (irrelevant data) and reducing its accuracy.[32] [33] A final drawback to neural networks is that the development model is empirical and because it is a new technique methodological problems remain.[32] In a direct comparison between neural networks and logistic regression models Tu and colleagues concluded that neural networks were better for predicting outcomes but that logistic regression was preferable when looking for possible causal relations between independent and dependent variables or when trying to understand the effect of predictor variables on an outcome.[32]

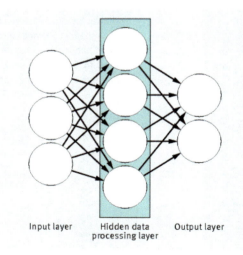

Fig 3 Schematic representation of an artificial neural network. The first column (input layer) represents a piece of data that can be put in to the neural network programme. The circles in the second column (hidden layer) represent the neural network programme assigned weight or numerical significance of each piece of data entered in the input layer. The final column (output layer) represents the dichotomous predicted outcome for the information entered

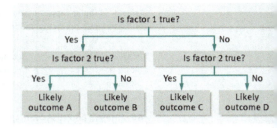

Fig 4 Simplified representation of a basic decision tree

Decision trees (CART analysis)

Classification and regression tree (CART) analysis uses non parametric tests to evaluate data and progressively divide it into subgroups based on the predictive independent variables.[4] The variables and discriminatory values used and the order in which the splitting occurs are produced by the underlying mathematical algorithm and are calculated to maximise the resulting predictive accuracy.[4] CART analysis produces "decision trees," which are generally easily understood and consequently translate well into everyday clinical practice (fig 4). By following the arrows indicated by the answers to each of the questions in the boxes clinicians will be directed to the predicted outcome for the patient. Examples of CARTs used in clinical practice include those to predict large oesophageal varices in cirrhotic patients and to predict the likelihood of hospital admission in patients with asthma.[36] [37] However, the CART model of prediction can be significantly less accurate than other models.[28] [38] This may be because the "leaves" on the trees contain too little data to be able to predict outcomes reliably.[3]

Conclusion

Each of the five main models has advantages and disadvantages, and no single model of prediction has been clearly shown to be superior to the others in all applications. As pressure on their time increases, doctors will need to become familiar with decision making tools and the statistical principles underlying them.

Contributors: STA wrote the original manuscript and subsequent revisions. He is the guarantor. SHL provided critical evaluation of the original manuscript, suggested revisions, and gave final approval for submission of the paper for consideration for publication.

Competing interests: All authors have completed the unified disclosure form at www.icmje.org/coi_disclosure.pdf (available on request from the corresponding author) and declare no support from any organisation for the submitted work; no financial relationships with any organisations that might have an interest in the submitted work in the past three years; and no other relationships or activities that could appear to have influenced the submitted work.

Provenance and peer review: Not commissioned; externally peer reviewed.

1   Toll DB, Janssen KJ, Vergouwe Y, Moons KG. Validation, updating and impact of clinical prediction rules: a review. *J Clin Epidemiol* 2008;61:1085-94.

2   Cook CE. Potential pitfalls of clinical prediction rules. *J Man Manip Ther* 2008;16:69-71.

3   Bellazzi R, Zupan B. Predictive data mining in clinical medicine: current issues and guidelines. *Int J Med Inform* 2008;77:81-97.

4   Grobman WA, Stamilio DM. Methods of clinical prediction. *Am J Obstet Gynecol* 2006;194:888-94.

5   Braitman LE, Davidoff F. Predicting clinical states in individual patients. *Ann Intern Med* 1996;125:406-12.

6   Altman DG, Bland JM. Diagnostic tests. 1: sensitivity and specificity. *BMJ* 1994;308:1552.

7   Altman DG, Bland JM. Diagnostic tests 2: predictive values. *BMJ* 1994;309:102.

8   Collins JA. Associate editor's commentary: mathematical modelling and clinical prediction. *Hum Reprod* 2005;20:2932-4.

9   Altman DG, Bland JM. Diagnostic tests 3: receiver operating characteristic plots. *BMJ* 1994;309:188.

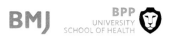

10   Reilly BM, Evans AT. Translating clinical research into clinical practice: impact of using prediction rules to make decisions. *Ann Intern Med* 2006;144:201-9.

11   Yealy DM, Auble TE. Choosing between clinical prediction rules. *N Engl J Med* 2003;349:2553-5.

12   Verma S, Hamilton K, Hawkins HH, Kothari R, Singal B, Buncher R, et al. Clinical application of the Ottawa ankle rules for the use of radiography in acute ankle injuries: an independent site assessment. *AJR Am J Roentgenol* 1997;169:825-7.

13   Kleinmuntz B. Why we still use our heads instead of formulas: toward an integrative approach. *Psychol Bull* 1990;107:296-310.

14   Marchese MC. Clinical versus actuarial prediction: a review of the literature. *Percept Mot Skills* 1992;75:583-94.

15   Bland JM, Altman DG. Statistics notes: validating scales and indexes. *BMJ* 2002;324:606-7.

16   Cookson J. A critique of the specialty certificate examinations of the Federation of Royal Colleges of Physicians of the UK. *Clin Med* 2010;10:141-4.

17   Liao L, Mark DB. Clinical prediction models: are we building better mousetraps? *J Am Coll Cardiol* 2003;42:851-3.

18   Gandara E, Wells PS. Diagnosis: use of clinical probability algorithms. *Clin Chest Med* 2010;31:629-39.

19   Bandiera G, Stiell IG, Wells GA, Clement C, De Maio V, Vandemheen KL, et al. The Canadian C-spine rule performs better than unstructured physician judgment. *Ann Emerg Med* 2003;42:395-402.

20   Gardner W, Lidz CW, Mulvey EP, Shaw EC. Clinical versus actuarial predictions of violence of patients with mental illnesses. *J Consult Clin Psychol* 1996;64:602-9.

21   Grove WM, Zald DH, Lebow BS, Snitz BE, Nelson C. Clinical versus mechanical prediction: a meta-analysis. *Psychol Assess* 2000;12:19-30.

22   Stiell IG, Clement CM, McKnight RD, Brison R, Schull MJ, Rowe BH, et al. The Canadian C-spine rule versus the NEXUS low-risk criteria in patients with trauma. *N Engl J Med* 2003;349:2510-8.

23   Alvarado A. A practical score for the early diagnosis of acute appendicitis. *Ann Emerg Med* 1986;15:557-64.

24   Taylor SL, Morgan DL, Denson KD, Lane MM, Pennington LR. A comparison of the Ranson, Glasgow, and APACHE II scoring systems to a multiple organ system score in predicting patient outcome in pancreatitis. *Am J Surg* 2005;189:219-22.

25   Bland JM, Altman DG. Statistics notes. The odds ratio. *BMJ* 2000;320:1468.

26   Doerfler R. On jargon: the lost art of nomography. *UMAP* 2009;30:457-93.

27   Siggaard-Andersen O. The acid-base status of the blood. *Scand J Clin Lab Invest* 1963;15(suppl 70):1-134.

28   Chun FK, Karakiewicz PI, Briganti A, Walz J, Kattan MW, Huland H, et al. A critical appraisal of logistic regression-based nomograms, artificial neural networks, classification and regression-tree models, look-up tables and risk-group stratification models for prostate cancer. *BJU Int* 2007;99:794-800.

29   Eastham JA, May R, Robertson JL, Sartor O, Kattan MW. Development of a nomogram that predicts the probability of a positive prostate biopsy in men with an abnormal digital rectal examination and a prostate-specific antigen between 0 and 4 ng/mL. *Urology* 1999;54:709-13.

30   Lam KK, Pang SC, Allan WG, Hill LE, Snell NJ, Fayers PM, et al. Predictive nomograms for forced expiratory volume, forced vital capacity, and peak expiratory flow rate, in Chinese adults and children. *Br J Dis Chest* 1983;77:390-6.

31   Neuro AI. Intelligent systems and neural networks. 2007. www.learnartificialneuralnetworks.com/.

32   Tu JV. Advantages and disadvantages of using artificial neural networks versus logistic regression for predicting medical outcomes. *J Clin Epidemiol* 1996;49:1225-31.

33   Ayer T, Chhatwal J, Alagoz O, Kahn CE Jr, Woods RW, Burnside ES. Informatics in radiology: comparison of logistic regression and artificial neural network models in breast cancer risk estimation. *Radiographics* 2009;30:13-22.

34   Westreich D, Lessler J, Funk MJ. Propensity score estimation: neural networks, support vector machines, decision trees (CART), and meta-classifiers as alternatives to logistic regression. *J Clin Epidemiol* 2010;63:826-33.

35   Hermundstad AM, Brown KS, Bassett DS, Carlson JM. Learning, memory, and the role of neural network architecture. *PLoS Comput Biol* 2010;7:e1002063.

36   Hong WD, Dong LM, Jiang ZC, Zhu QH, Jin SQ. Prediction of large esophageal varices in cirrhotic patients using classification and regression tree analysis. *Clinics (Sao Paulo)* 2011;66:119-24.

37   Tsai CL, Clark S, Camargo CA Jr. Risk stratification for hospitalization in acute asthma: the CHOP classification tree. *Am J Emerg Med* 2010;28:803-8.

38   Austin PC, Tu JV, Lee DS. Logistic regression had superior performance compared with regression trees for predicting in-hospital mortality in patients hospitalized with heart failure. *J Clin Epidemiol* 2010;63:1145-55.

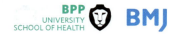

When is a further clinical trial justified?

Manuela L Ferreira, research fellow[1], Robert D Herbert, professor[2],
Michael J Crowther, research associate[3], Arianne Verhagen, associate professor[4],
Alex J Sutton, professor of medical statistics[3]

[1]The George Institute for Global Health, University of Sydney, PO Box M201, Missenden Road, NSW 2050, Australia

[2]Neuroscience Research Australia, Sydney, Australia

[3]Department of Health Sciences, University of Leicester, UK

[4]Department of General Practice, Erasmus Medical Centre University, Rotterdam, Netherlands

Correspondence to: M L Ferreira
mferreira@georgeinstitute.org.au

Cite this as: BMJ 2012;345:e5913

DOI: 10.1136/bmj.e5913

http://www.bmj.com/content/345/bmj.e5913

Even on their own the best randomised trials do not usually provide convincing evidence of the effectiveness (or lack of effectiveness) of an intervention. Consensus about effectiveness is usually only achieved when a meta-analysis of several high quality trials shows a statistically significant effect. Until such a consensus is achieved researchers may claim that a new trial is justified. We will refer to this as the "conventional approach" to justification of a new trial.

Two problems, and solutions

There are two problems with the conventional approach. The first concerns the interpretation of existing evidence: interpretation of data from clinical trials or meta-analyses is reduced to a decision about whether the intervention is "effective" or "ineffective."[1] The simplistic classification of interventions as effective or ineffective fails to make the important distinction between interventions that have trivial effects and those that have worthwhile effects.

A health intervention produces "worthwhile" effects when it does more good than harm. Here we must use the term "harm" to include all of the negative aspects of interventions: from a patient's perspective, these could include risks of adverse events, pain or discomfort, cost, or inconvenience. The role of clinical trials is to provide unbiased estimates of the beneficial effects of health interventions so that it can be ascertained whether those effects outweigh risks, costs, and inconvenience.

Several methods have been developed to determine what beneficial effect would outweigh the risks, costs, and inconvenience of an intervention. In a recent review we argued such methods should be based on patients' (usually not researchers' or clinicians') perceptions, intervention specific, and expressed in terms of differences between outcomes with and without intervention.[2] One method potentially satisfies all three criteria. The "benefit-harm trade-off method" involves presenting patients with hypothetical scenarios about the effects of an intervention and identifying the smallest hypothetical effect for which the patient would choose to receive the intervention.[3] We refer to this as the "smallest worthwhile effect" of intervention to differentiate it from similar constructs such as the "minimum clinically important difference" derived with alternative methods.

Figure 1 illustrates how information about the smallest worthwhile effect of an intervention can be used to interpret an estimate of the effect of intervention from a

ABSTRACT

High quality randomised trials provide unbiased estimate of the effects of health interventions, but the findings of a single trial are rarely conclusive. Usually data from several similar trials must be pooled together to draw firm conclusions about the effectiveness of an intervention. This article considers how to determine whether data from existing trials are conclusive and, if not, whether a further trial is justified.

meta-analysis (or, for that matter, from an individual clin trial). The figure shows six hypothetical pooled estima of the effect of a health intervention (A-F) obtained f six hypothetical meta-analyses of randomised trials. magnitude of the pooled estimate of effect is indicated the location of the diamonds along the horizontal axis. meta-analyses in which the effect is quantified as a m difference in outcomes of treated and control groups example, weighted mean difference or standardised m difference) the line of no effect would have a value of 0. meta-analyses in which the effect is quantified as a r of outcomes of treated and control groups (for exam relative risk, odds ratio, hazard ratio, or incidence rate ra the line of no effect would have a value of 1. For e possible outcome, the statistical significance of a test the null hypothesis (that is, no effect of intervention shown, along with an interpretation of the outcome ba on consideration of the estimated size of the effect.

In each of the six scenarios one of three conclusions be drawn: the effect is worth while (outcome F in fig 1 is unclear if the effect is worth while (outcomes D and or the effect is not worth while (outcomes A, B, and C further trial is only justified when it is unclear if the ef is worth while. Note that the statistical significance of a of the null hypothesis is not relevant when determinin a further trial is justified. Further trials should only be d in scenarios D and E.

A second problem with the conventional appro to determining whether a further trial is justified is t the decision is often made without consideration of h the findings of the new trial might contribute to exist evidence.[4] Usually it will be an updated meta-analysis of trial data, not just the data from the new trial, that provi the most precise estimate of effect of intervention. A furt trial is only justified when addition of data from the n trial to a meta-analysis of existing trials could conv uncertainty about whether the effects of intervention worthwhile (outcomes D and E in fig 1) to the conclus that the intervention is worth while (outcome F) or is worthwhile (outcomes A-C).

It is widely believed that provided a clinical trial is la enough it will confer a high degree of certainty about effects of intervention. (Here we put aside important issu about risk of bias and quality of interventions.) A surpris new idea is that sometimes no trial of any size, when add to an existing random effects meta-analysis, will be a

SUMMARY POINTS

- A further clinical trial may be justified when the existing evidence from high quality clinical trials does not clearly indicate whether an intervention is or is not worth while
- Benefit-harm trade-off studies can determine what constitutes a "worthwhile" effect
- When a meta-analysis of existing trials does not provide clear findings about whether an intervention has worthwhile effects, and a further trial is being considered, extended funnel plots can be used to explore the potential impact of a new trial on the updated meta-analysis
- These procedures can be used to determine if a further clinical trial is justified

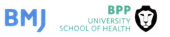

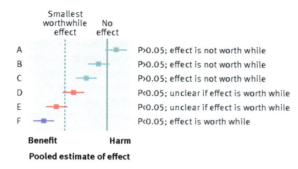

Fig 1 Interpretation of six pooled estimates of effect from six hypothetical meta-analyses of randomised trials. Error bars are 95% confidence intervals

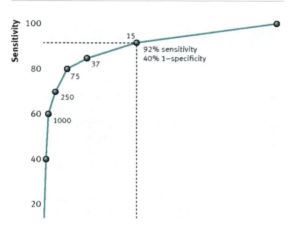

Fig 2 Forest plot showing estimates of effect of exercise on chronic low back pain. Summary data (mean effect, expressed as a difference between treated and control groups) from eight randomised trials (squares) with pooled estimate from random effects meta-analysis (diamond). Values less than 0 are indicative of a beneficial effect (reduction in pain). Error bars are 95% confidence intervals. Two values for the smallest worthwhile effect are shown, corresponding, respectively, to the 50th and 80th centiles of estimates of the smallest worthwhile effect obtained in a benefit harm trade-off study

to provide a high degree of certainty about the effects of intervention.[4] This is because when the findings of the new trial are sufficiently extreme to have a noticeable effect on the pooled estimate of effect, they may increase between trial heterogeneity to the extent that the data from the new trial increase, rather than decrease, the width of the confidence interval about the pooled estimate of effect (see supplementary file).

Two of the authors have developed methods for evaluating whether it is plausible that a new trial could convert existing uncertainty about the effects of intervention into clear evidence for or against the existence of a worthwhile effect.[4 5] These methods include "extended funnel plots"—graphical augmentations of the funnel plots traditionally used to investigate small study bias in meta-analysis.[6 7] The shaded contours of an extended funnel plot show how the conclusions of an updated meta-analysis can be influenced by the findings and size of the new trial: particular combinations of trial findings and trial sizes may result in the conclusion that the effect of intervention is clearly worth while, or clearly not worth while, or remains uncertain. Extended funnel plots can be constructed using the extfunnel macro in Stata.[6]

In the following section we briefly illustrate the use of benefit-harm trade-off studies and extended funnel plots to determine whether a further trial is justified. The example of exercise for chronic low back pain is used. We focus on

the short term effects of exercise on pain, measured on a 100 point scale.

The smallest worthwhile effect of exercise for chronic back pain

Using the benefit-harm trade-off method we obtained estimates of the smallest worthwhile effect of exercise for chronic low back pain. We ranked the smallest worthwhile effects reported by 95 participants and calculated the 50th and 80th centiles—that is, the effects considered large enough to be worth while by 50% and 80% of participants. On the 100 point pain scale the 50th and 80th centiles corresponded to treatment effects of 20 and 30 points, respectively.

Existing evidence of the effect of exercise on chronic back pain

We used optimised search strategies to update to August 2011 a recent meta-analysis of the effects of exercise on chronic low back pain.[8] Pain data were rescaled to a common 0-100 scale. Data from eight trials[9 10 11 12 13 14 15] were pooled in a random effects meta-analysis (fig 2). These analyses showed that compared with no treatment, exercise reduces pain on average by 14 points (95% confidence interval 6 to 21 points) on a 100 point scale. The effect is clearly significant (P of test of no effect <0.001), but the more interesting issue concerns whether the effect is large enough to be worth while.

Does exercise produce worthwhile reductions in chronic back pain?

Use of the 80th centile of the smallest worthwhile effect (a 30 point reduction in pain) might be justified if it was believed that the interpretation of clinical trials should be based on an effect of intervention considered to be worth while by most people in the population of interest. As fig 2 shows, if the 80th centile is used, one would conclude that exercise is clearly not worth while for treatment of chronic back pain (because the confidence interval for the effect of exercise only includes effects <30). In that case there would be no need to do a further trial.

Alternatively, use of the 50th centile of the smallest worthwhile effect (a 20 point reduction in pain) might be justified if it was believed that the interpretation of clinical trials should be based on effects considered to be worth while by typical people in the population of interest. As fig 2 shows, if the 50th centile is used, it is not clear whether exercise is worth while for treatment of chronic back pain because the confidence interval for the effect of exercise includes values above and below 20.

The 50th centile (the median) of the smallest worthwhile effect may be more justifiable as it may be particularly important to determine if the expected effect of intervention is of interest to a typical person in the population of interest. Consequently we concluded it is not clear if exercise has worthwhile effects on chronic back pain and we considered whether a new trial could resolve this uncertainty.

What influence would the findings of a new trial have?

Figure 3A is an extended funnel plot showing the potential conclusions arising from a new trial of exercise for chronic back pain. In fig 3B the plot has been modified so that the sample size, rather than the standard error, is shown on the vertical axis. In both panels the horizontal axis represents the size of the effect of intervention that could be observed in a new trial. The horizontal axis has been drawn so that its

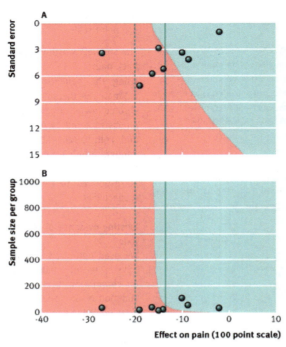

Fig 3 Extended funnel plots showing the predicted consequences of a further trial on the updated conclusions of a meta-analysis of the effects of exercise for back pain

extremes are the limits of the 95% prediction interval.[16] (The prediction interval is the range of effects that is predicted could occur in a new trial, given the effects observed in the eight existing trials.) The vertical axis reflects the size of the trial. In fig 3A the size of the new trial is expressed in terms of its standard error. In fig 3B the size of the trial is expressed as the number of participants in the trial. (Here it is assumed the standard deviation is known—it was assigned a value of 15—and that there will be two equally sized groups.) Data from the existing meta-analysis (fig 2) have been superimposed on the extended funnel plots (same data in both panels). The mean effects from each of the eight randomised trials are shown as circles, the solid vertical line is the pooled estimate of the mean effect of exercise for chronic back pain, and the dashed line is the smallest worthwhile effect. A new trial could produce a finding that is located anywhere on the plot—the location in the horizontal direction depends on the estimate of effect provided by the new trial and the location in the vertical direction depends on the size of the new trial. Each point on the plot is coloured red or blue to indicate the conclusion that would be drawn from the updated meta-analysis if the new trial had that particular combination of effect size (horizontal axis) and trial size (vertical axis). The colour codes are the same as in fig 1. Thus these plots show that if the findings of a new trial of exercise for chronic back pain were to be added to the existing meta-analysis, the updated conclusion of the meta-analysis could be that the effect of exercise is too small to be worth while (blue regions) or that it is uncertain if the effect is worth while (red regions). There are no purple regions on the plot, indicating that it is unlikely a new trial could show that exercise has a worthwhile effect.

Although the extended funnel plot indicates there is no real possibility a new trial could show that exercise produces worthwhile reductions in chronic back pain, some clinical trialists might none the less consider carrying out a further trial to determine if exercise does not have worthwhile effects. (It would be useful to know if this were true as

exercise is currently used widely for the management chronic back pain.) However, sample size calculation (supplementary file) suggest that this may be futile: w a sample size of 500 there is only a 55% probability of t updated meta-analysis concluding that exercise does n produce worthwhile effects and a 45% chance of concludi ongoing uncertainty. Note that conventional pow calculations[17] would conclude very differently: they wou suggest that a new trial with 500 participants would ha a power of nearly 100% to detect the smallest worthwh effect.

In summary, while existing trials clearly show statistica significant effects of exercise for chronic back pain, th neither confirm nor rule out the possibility that exerci has worthwhile effects; and it is likely that a new trial, ev a large trial, would not resolve uncertainty about wheth the effects are large enough to be worth while. The latt conclusion is based on consideration of the contributi of just one new trial. We acknowledge that several tri (perhaps even several small trials) may yield certain where one large trial does not.[4] Alternatively, it may possible to use individual patient data meta-analyses metaregression methods to explain some of the betwe trial heterogeneity. An additional consideration may be t cost of a new trial. A complete justification of a new tr would weigh the cost of the trial against the value of t information it generates.[18]

The methods we have described can be based on eith fixed effect or random effects meta-analyses. We recomme routine use of random effects meta-analysis. Wh heterogeneity is present, however, random effects mode limit the impact of any individual study.[4] A consequence that in some circumstances, as in the example used her new studies can have little impact on existing conclusion

Conclusions

This article has described the use of benefit-harm studies define the smallest worthwhile effect of intervention, a the use of extended funnel plots to explore the potenti influence of a new trial on the findings of an updat meta-analysis. Clinical trialists should consider using the procedures when deciding whether to carry out a furth clinical trial. Peer reviewers and granting bodies could se evidence from these sorts of analyses when assessi requests for funding to conduct a further trial.[4 19]

Contributors: MLF, RDH, and AV conceived the idea for the study. M and RDH are guarantors. MLF carried out the literature search, data extraction, and benefit-harm trade-off study. MJC and AJS developed the extended funnel plot methods. MJC, AJS, and RDH carried out th extended funnel plot analysis. MLF and RDH wrote the first draft of the manuscript. All authors made substantial contributions to the final manuscript.

Funding: MJC is funded by a National Institute for Health Research Methods Fellowship (RP-PG-0407-10314). RDH is supported by an NHMRC research fellowship.

Competing interests: All authors have completed the ICMJE uniform disclosure form at www.icmje.org/coi_disclosure.pdf (available on request from the corresponding author) and declare: no support fro any organisation for the submitted work; no financial relationships with any organisations that might have an interest in the submitted work in the previous three years; and no other relationships or activities that could appear to have influenced the submitted work.

Provenance and peer review: Not commissioned; externally peer reviewed.

1   Silva-Aycaguer LC, Suarez-Gil P, Fernandez-Somoano A. The null hypothesis significance test in health sciences research (1995-2006) statistical analysis and interpretation. *BMC Med Res Methodol* 2010;10:44.
2   Ferreira ML, Herbert RD, Ferreira PH, Latimer J, Ostelo RW, Nasciment DP, et al. A critical review of methods used to determine the smalle

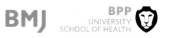

worthwhile effect of interventions for low back pain. *J Clin Epidemiol* 2012;65:253-61.

3   Barrett B, Brown R, Mundt M, Dye L, Alt J, Safdar N, et al. Using benefit harm tradeoffs to estimate sufficiently important difference: the case of the common cold. *Med Decis Making* 2005;25:47-55.

4   Sutton AJ, Cooper NJ, Jones DR, Lambert PC, Thompson JR, Abrams KR. Evidence-based sample size calculations based upon updated meta-analysis. *Stat Med* 2007;26:2479-500.

5   Sutton AJ, Cooper NJ, Jones DR. Evidence synthesis as the key to more coherent and efficient research. *BMC Med Res Methodol* 2009;9:29.

6   Langan D, Higgins JP, Gregory W, Sutton AJ. Graphical augmentations to the funnel plot assess the impact of additional evidence on a meta-analysis. *J Clin Epidemiol* 2012;65:511-9.

7   Crowther M, Langan D, Sutton A. Graphical augmentations to the funnel plot to assess the impact of a new study on an existing meta-analysis. *Stata J* 2012;(In press).

8   Ferreira ML, Smeets RJ, Kamper SJ, Ferreira PH, Machado LA. Can we explain heterogeneity among randomized clinical trials of exercise for chronic back pain? A meta-regression analysis of randomized controlled trials. *Phys Ther* 2010;90:1383-403.

9   Albaladejo C, Kovacs FM, Royuela A, del Pino R, Zamora J. The efficacy of a short education program and a short physiotherapy program for treating low back pain in primary care: a cluster randomized trial. *Spine* 2010;35:483-96.

10 Bakhtiary AH, Safavi-Farokhi Z, Aminian-Far A. Influence of vibration on delayed onset of muscle soreness following eccentric exercise. *Br J Sports Med* 2007;41:145-8.

11 Djavid GE, Mehrdad R, Ghasemi M, Hasan-Zadeh H, Sotoodeh-Manesh A, Pouryaghoub G. In chronic low back pain, low level laser therapy combined with exercise is more beneficial than exercise alone in the long term: a randomised trial. *Aust J Physiother* 2007;53:155-60.

12 Kell RT, Asmundson GJ. A comparison of two forms of periodized exercise rehabilitation programs in the management of chronic nonspecific low-back pain. *J Strength Cond Res* 2009;23:513-23.

13 Kofotolis N, Kellis E. Effects of two 4-week proprioceptive neuromuscular facilitation programs on muscle endurance, flexibility, and functional performance in women with chronic low back pain. *Phys Ther* 2006;86:1001-12.

14 Saper RB, Sherman KJ, Cullum-Dugan D, Davis RB, Phillips RS, Culpepper L. Yoga for chronic low back pain in a predominantly minority population: a pilot randomized controlled trial. *Altern Ther Health Med* 2009;15:18-27.

15 Smeets RJ, Vlaeyen JW, Hidding A, Kester AD, van der Heijden GJ, Knottnerus JA. Chronic low back pain: physical training, graded activity with problem solving training, or both? The one-year post-treatment results of a randomized controlled trial. *Pain* 2008;134:263-76.

16 Riley RD, Higgins JP, Deeks JJ. Interpretation of random effects meta-analyses. *BMJ* 2011;342:d549.

17 Julious S. Sample sizes for clinical trials with Normal data. *Stat Med* 2004;23:1921-86.

18 Willan AR, Pinto EM. The value of information and optimal clinical trial design. *Stat Med* 2005;24:1791-806.

19 Higgins JP, Thompson SG, Spiegelhalter DJ. A re-evaluation of random-effects meta-analysis. *J R Stat Soc Ser A Stat Soc* 2009;172:137-59.

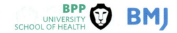

Out of sight but not out of mind: how to search for unpublished clinical trial evidence

An-Wen Chan, assistant professor and Phelan scientist

Women's College Research
Institute, University of Toronto,
Toronto, Ontario, Canada

Corrrespondence to: A-W Chan
anwen.chan@utoronto.ca

Cite this as: *BMJ* 2012;344:d8013

DOI: 10.1136/bmj.d8013

http://www.bmj.com/content/344/
bmj.d8013

Systematic reviews of randomised wtrials play a key role in guiding patient care and health policy. Their validity depends to a large extent on reviewers' ability to retrieve relevant information from all existing trials. Unfortunately, about half of clinical trials remain unpublished after receiving ethics approval—particularly those with statistically non-significant findings.[1] Even when published, most journal articles do not report all of the outcome data or key methodological information.[2][3] The overall result is that the published literature tends to overestimate the efficacy and underestimate the harms of a given intervention, while providing insufficient information for readers to evaluate the risk of bias.

It is thus important that systematic reviewers adopt a comprehensive strategy to search beyond the published literature. The optimal systematic review would have complete information about every trial—the full protocol, final study report, raw dataset, and any journal publications and regulatory submissions.[4] The eligibility and risk of bias for each trial could then be evaluated, regardless of its publication status.

There are several potential sources of unpublished information on trial methods and results (table). These sources can help to identify the existence and results of unpublished trials, as well as unreported outcomes within published trials. They can also provide methodological information that facilitates assessment of risk of bias, including the detection of discrepancies between unpublished and published methods.[5][6] Systematic reviewers should consider using all potential information sources as part of their search strategy, while keeping in mind the strengths and limitations of each source (table).

Trial registries and results databases

Trial registries serve as a readily accessible online resource for identifying unpublished trials and unreported outcomes. Since 2005, prospective trial registration has gained broad acceptance as an important means of enhancing transparency and tracking the existence of clinical trials at inception. Key stakeholders—including medical journal editors, legislators, and funding agencies—provide enforcement mechanisms that have greatly improved adherence to registration practices.

Basic protocol information on ongoing and completed trials of any intervention type can be retrieved via the World Health Organization's International Clinical Trials Registry Platform Search Portal (www.who.int/trialsearch/).

ABSTRACT

A key challenge in conducting systematic reviews is to identify the existence and results of unpublished trials, and unreported methods and outcomes within published trials. **An-Wen Chan** provides guidance for reviewers on adopting a comprehensive strategy to search beyond the published literature

This searches records from national and international registries that meet certain standards, including W Primary Registries and ClinicalTrials.gov. Users can sea the main registry fields using key words related to study topic, sponsor, recruitment status, and sites. W the same trial is registered in multiple registries, the W Search Portal displays similar records together to facili identification of duplicate records. Some registry webs also provide access to the history of changes to registered information fields.

In addition to basic protocol information, certain regist house study results. Since 2008, ClinicalTrials.gov has the legislative mandate to record summary results for tr (other than phase I) that involve a drug or device regula by the US Food and Drug Administration.[7] Sponsors required by law to provide summary baseline and outco data, which are displayed in a standard format.

Some pharmaceutical companies also maintain their voluntary trial registers and results databases for drugs have received regulatory approval. Systematic reviews h previously incorporated unpublished data retrieved fi industry registers.[8] These public registers provide a syno of trial methods and summary results as dictated company policy. Information is presented in various form with non-standardised content. For certain companies, th may be information posted for older trials of some marke interventions. It should be noted that ClinicalStudyResu org, the results database launched by the Internatic Federation of Pharmaceutical Manufacturers and Associati in 2004, was to be discontinued by the end of 2011 beca of overlap with other registries.

Beyond basic protocol information and results, registries have the potential to be the repository for protocols. Legislation in the US allows for the possibility requiring submission of full protocols to ClinicalTrials. for applicable trials.[7] Furthermore, certain pharmaceut companies are recognising the importance of public acc to full protocols and have committed to posting them their register for all published trials.[9] These are promis first steps towards facilitating access to protocols for trials, regardless of publication status.

Despite their importance, trial registries and resi databases have several limitations. Firstly, there is universal mechanism for ensuring adherence to standa for registration or results disclosure, meaning that not trials will be captured. Journal policy will be ineffective trials that are not intended for publication, while curr legislation does not pertain to procedural, education

SUMMARY POINTS

- The validity of systematic reviews relies on the identification of all relevant evidence
- Systematic reviewers should search for unpublished information on the methods and results of published and unpublished clinical trials
- The potential sources of unpublished information on clinical trials have expanded over recent years
- Recognition of the strengths and limitations of these key information sources can help to identify areas for further emphasis and improvement

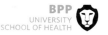

Table Potential sources of unpublished information on trial methods and results

Source	Potential information	Strengths	Limitations
Trial registries (non-industry)	Methods: BasicResults: Summary	Broad scope of trials (ongoing, completed, any intervention) Standardised core content Free accessibility Searchability Audit trail of changes to registry entries Potential posting of full protocols	Lack of universal adherence mechanism Variable quality of information Limited methodological information Limited availability before 2005
Results database (ClinicalTrials.gov)	Methods: Basic Results: Summary	Standard format and content Legislative enforcement for applicable trials	Lack of universal adherence mechanism Limited availability before 2008
Trial registries and results databases (industry)	Methods: Basic Results: Summary	Free accessibility Searchability Potential posting of full protocols Availability of older trials for select drugs	Limited to marketed drugs Lack of external oversight Variable format, quality, and content
Regulatory agency online databases	Methods: Basic Results: Summary	Availability of all trials for most approved drugs Database searchability Disclosure supported by legislation	Variable format and content Redacted content Limited methodological information Limited to drug trials
Regulatory agency submissions (on request)	Methods: Full protocol Results: Clinical study report	Availability of all trials for approved drugs and devices Detailed methods and results Disclosure supported by legislation	Potential for lengthy delays Request may be rejected Redacted content Limited to drug and device trials
Trialist and sponsor contact	Methods: Full protocol Results: Variable	Detailed methods and results Opportunity to correspond about specific issues	Burdensome Variable response rates
Litigation documents	Methods: Full protocol Results: Clinical study report	Detailed methods and results	Request may be rejected Unclear accessibility for external researchers
Conference abstracts	Methods: Basic Results: Limited	Not restricted by intervention type	Difficult to find Limited methodological information and results
Internet search	Methods: Full protocol Results: Not applicable	Ease of use Short completion time	Variable yield

and other unregulated interventions. Secondly, the quality of registered information is highly variable and often uninformative.[7] [10] [11] [12] [13] Changes to registered information are common,[12] meaning that systematic reviewers should review the history of amendments for each registry record. Thirdly, even when a trial is fully registered with complete summary results presented, there is a limited amount of methodological information available that is largely inadequate for assessing the risk of bias.[10] This concern would be addressed if full protocols were made available on the registries.[9] [14] Finally, most trials will not have been registered prior to the introduction of International Committee of Medical Journal Editors policy and WHO standards in 2005.

Regulatory agencies

Regulatory agencies have access to substantially more clinical trial information than the healthcare providers, patients, and researchers who use and evaluate the interventions. Successful attempts to obtain access to regulatory data have previously necessitated litigation and incurred lengthy delays.[15] [16] [17] Over recent years, regulatory agencies have recognised the need to address this untenable situation by increasing public access to information from regulatory submissions.[18] [19]

There are currently two main routes for reviewers to obtain trial data from regulatory agencies—scientific reviews posted in online databases,[20] [21] and written requests to regulatory agencies.[15] Scientific reviews of regulatory submissions contain a narrative summary of the clinical trials that form the basis for approval of regulated drugs. These documents are generally available on searchable internet databases provided by the US Food and Drug Administration and the European Medicines Agency:

- Drugs@FDA — www.accessdata.fda.gov/scripts/cder/drugsatfda/index.cfm

- European public assessment reports (EPAR)—www.ema.europa.eu/ema/index.jsp?curl=pages/medicines/landing/epar_search.jsp&murl=menus/medicines/medicines.jsp&mid=WC0b01ac058001d125&jsenabled=true

Relevant clinical trial summaries are generally labelled as "Statistical review" on Drugs@FDA, and "Scientific Discussion" in EPAR. The Pharmaceuticals and Medical Devices Agency in Japan (http://www.pmda.go.jp/english/service/approved.html) also posts a limited number of reviews with English translations for select drugs and devices.

Limitations of the scientific reviews obtained from regulatory agency websites include the variable presentation format and the lack of text search facility for some scanned documents. In addition, the content is not standardised, information deemed to be commercially sensitive is redacted, and insufficient methodological detail is provided to assess the risk of bias for a trial. Furthermore, many trials are not included in regulatory databases, such as trials of devices and non-regulated interventions. Most trials conducted after regulatory approval would not be captured. For the European Medicines Agency, drugs that are approved by regulators in individual countries but not the central agency will not have public assessment reports available. Drugs@FDA includes information on withdrawn drugs but does not provide scientific reviews for unapproved drugs or drugs approved before 1998.

A second approach has the potential to yield more detailed information from regulatory agencies. Reviewers can make written requests to access the trial protocols and detailed clinical study reports submitted by sponsors.

As of December 2010, the European Medicines Agency has committed to accommodating such requests for documents contained in regulatory submissions for drugs, subject to redaction of commercially sensitive information.[19] This important advance will be expanded in the future to include proactive public disclosure of documents on the European Medicines Agency website as part of routine practice. The US Food and Drug Administration has previously granted access to clinical trial documents in response to litigation relating to freedom of information requests[16][17] and is also exploring ways to increase transparency.[18]

Limitations of this second approach include potentially lengthy delays in receiving a final decision from regulators, resource-intensive appeals or litigation for denied requests, redaction of potentially important information from documents, and lack of information on interventions other than regulated drugs and devices.

Contacting trialists and sponsors

Systematic reviewers have had variable success in contacting trialists, clinicians, and sponsors for information about unpublished trials.[4][22][23][24][25] Efforts to obtain full trial protocols from trialists have been largely disappointing.[26][27] On the other hand, surveys soliciting information on the existence and statistical significance of unreported outcomes for published trials have had higher response rates from trialists.[28][29] These surveys have also yielded information about the reasons for changing or omitting trial outcomes.

Logistical obstacles include the burden of identifying up to date contact information and sending inquiries and reminders to a potentially large number of individuals who might have knowledge about existing trials. It is also likely that trials for which additional information is provided by investigators or sponsors will differ systematically from trials without such information provided.

Systematic reviewers will need to weigh up the potential yield and costs of contacting investigators and sponsors, which will vary depending on the topic and scope of the review. At a minimum, for each trial identified in the systematic review, it would be reasonable for reviewers to contact investigators to request full protocols as well as information on unreported outcomes, unpublished trials, and other areas of potential bias.

Other sources of information

In some cases trial protocols and results can be obtained from litigation documents. Examples include researchers who had access to internal company documents while serving as expert witnesses in litigation against pharmaceutical companies.[30][31][32] In many jurisdictions, these documents are deemed confidential and their use is restricted to the purposes of the particular litigation—unless unsealed through a court order or agreement by the company. Systematic reviewers who are external to the litigation could submit a request to have the documents unsealed by the court to serve the public interest, although this approach has not been widely tested for pharmaceutical data. More extensive experience with public availability and archiving of litigation documents exists for other industries.[33]

Another potential source of information consists of conference abstracts.[34] The Cochrane handbook lists several databases of abstracts that can be useful to search.[35] Given the limited amount of information on trial methods and results contained in abstracts, their usefulness lies mainly with identifying the existence of a trial and the types of outcomes measured.

Finally, an internet search of key words can be done [to] locate full trial protocols in a relatively short amount [of] time. The median search time in one systematic review w[as] 12 minutes per trial, with protocols being found for five [of] 42 trials.[36] The retrieved documents are often those post[ed] on the websites of specific trials, trial groups, and funde[rs.]

Conclusions

Given the dangers of selective data suppression and bias[ed] study design or conduct, it is critical that systema[tic] reviewers search beyond the literature for additio[nal] information on both published and unpublished tria[ls.] The potential sources of information on study metho[ds] and results have expanded over recent years, particula[rly] for pharmaceutical trials. These sources can provi[de] complementary trial information that can be collated a[nd] compared to identify discrepancies and evaluate the ri[sk] of bias.

It is important to recognise the limitations and varia[ble] yield of existing information sources. Much work rema[ins] to ensure that comprehensive, high quality informati[on] is publicly available for all trials, including full protoco[ls,] clinical study reports, and raw datasets.[4][14][37] There is a[lso] a need to develop rigorous methods for reviewing the la[rge] amount of unpublished trial information that can potentia[lly] be retrieved.[4][15] Only with continued advances in access [to] clinical trial information can the systematic evaluation [of] health interventions become more accurate, efficient, a[nd] reliable for patient care.

Contributors: A-WC was responsible for interpretation of informatio[n,] drafting the article, and final approval of the version to be publishe[d.]

Competing interests: All authors have completed the Unified Competing Interest form at http://www.icmje.org/coi_disclosure.pdf (available on request from the corresponding author) and declare: no support from any organisation for the submitted work; no financial relationships with any organisations that might have a interest in the submitted work in the previous three years; no othe[r] relationships or activities that could appear to have influenced the submitted work."

Provenance and peer review: Commissioned; externally peer reviewed.

1   Song F, Parekh S, Hooper L, Loke YK, Ryder J, Sutton AJ, et al. Dissemination and publication of research findings: An updated review of related biases. Health Technol Assess 2010;14:1-193.
2   Dwan K, Altman DG, Arnaiz JA, Bloom J, Chan A-W, Cronin E, et al. Systematic review of the empirical evidence of study publication bi[as] and outcome reporting bias. PLoS One 2008;3:e3081.
3   Hopewell S, Dutton S, Yu LM, Chan A-W, Altman DG. The quality of reports of randomised trials in 2000 and 2006: comparative study o[f] articles indexed in PubMed. BMJ 2010;340:c723.
4   Jefferson T, Doshi P, Thompson M, Heneghan C. Ensuring safe and effective evidence for drugs—who can do what it takes? BMJ 2011;342:c7258.
5   Higgins JP, Altman DG, Gøtzsche PC, Jüni P, Moher D, Oxman AD, et al. The Cochrane Collaboration's tool for assessing risk of bias in randomised trials. BMJ 2011;343:d5928.
6   Chan A-W, Hróbjartsson A, Jørgensen KJ, Gøtzsche PC, Altman DG. Discrepancies in sample size calculations and data analyses reporte[d] in randomized trials: comparison of publications with protocols. BM[J] 2008;337:a2299.
7   Zarin DA, Tse T, Williams RJ, Califf RM, Ide NC. The ClinicalTrials. gov results database—update and key issues. N Engl J Med 2011;364:852-60.
8   Nissen SE, Wolski K. Effect of rosiglitazone on the risk of myocardial infarction and death from cardiovascular causes. N Engl J Med 2007;356:2457-71.
9   GlaxoSmithKline. Public disclosure of clinical research. Global Public Policy Issues, October 2011. Available from www.gsk.com/policies/GSK-on-disclosure-of-clinical-trial-information.pdf.
10 Reveiz L, Chan A-W, Krleža-Jerić K, Granados CE, Pinart M, Etxeandia I, et al. Reporting of methodologic information on trial registries for quality assessment: A study of trial records retrieved from the WHO search portal. PLoS ONE 2010;5:e12484.
11 Ross JS, Mulvey GK, Hines EM, Nissen SE, Krumholz HM. Trial publication after registration in ClinicalTrials.gov: a cross-sectional analysis. PLoS Med 2009;6:e1000144.

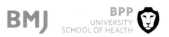

12 Huić M, Marušić M, Marušić A. Completeness and changes in registered data and reporting bias of randomized controlled trials in ICMJE journals after trial registration policy. *PLoS One* 2011;6:e25258.

13 Viergever RF, Ghersi D. The quality of registration of clinical trials. *PLoS One* 2011;6:e14701.

14 Chan A-W. Access to clinical trial data. *BMJ* 2011;342:d80.

15 Gøtzsche PC, Jørgensen AW. Opening up data at the European Medicines Agency. *BMJ* 2011;342:d2686.

16 Kesselheim AS, Mello MM. Confidentiality laws and secrecy in medical research: Improving public access to data on drug safety. *Health Aff (Millwood)* 2007;26:483-91.

17 Lurie P, Zieve A. Sometimes the silence can be like the thunder: Access to pharmaceutical data at the FDA. *Law Contemporary Problems* 2008;69:85-97.

18 Asamoah AK, Sharfstein JM. Transparency at the Food and Drug Administration. *N Engl J Med* 2010;362:2341-3.

19 European Medicines Agency. EMA/110196/2006. European Medicines Agency policy on access to documents (related to medicinal products for human and veterinary use), POLICY/0043. 2010.

20 Rising K, Bacchetti P, Bero L. Reporting bias in drug trials submitted to the food and drug administration: review of publication and presentation. *PLoS Med* 2008;5:e217.

21 Turner EH, Matthews AM, Linardatos E, Tell RA, Rosenthal R. Selective publication of antidepressant trials and its influence on apparent efficacy. *N Engl J Med* 2008;358:252-60.

22 Reveiz L, Cardona AF, Ospina EG, de Agular S. An e-mail survey identified unpublished studies for systematic reviews. *J Clin Epidemiol* 2006;59:755-8.

23 McGrath J, Davies G, Soares K. Writing to authors of systematic reviews elicited further data in 17% of cases. *BMJ* 1998;316:631.

24 Clarke M, Greaves L. Identifying relevant studies for systematic reviews. *BMJ* 1995;310:741.

25 Hetherington J, Dickersin K, Chalmers I, Meinert CL. Retrospective and prospective identification of unpublished controlled trials: lessons from a survey of obstetricians and pediatricians. *Pediatrics* 1989;84:374-80.

26 Smyth RM, Kirkham JJ, Jacoby A, Altman DG, Gamble C, Williamson PR. Frequency and reasons for outcome reporting bias in clinical trials: Interviews with trialists. *BMJ* 2011;342:c7153.

27 Hahn S, Williamson PR, Hutton JL. Investigation of within-study selective reporting in clinical research: follow-up of applications submitted to a local research ethics committee. *J Eval Clin Pract* 2002;8:353-9.

28 Chan A-W, Altman DG. Identifying outcome reporting bias in randomised trials on PubMed: review of publications and survey of authors. *BMJ* 2005;330:753.

29 Chan A-W, Hróbjartsson A, Haahr MT, Gøtzsche PC, Altman DG. Empirical evidence for selective reporting of outcomes in randomized trials: comparison of protocols to published articles. *JAMA* 2004;291:2457-65.

30 Vedula SS, Bero L, Scherer RW, Dickersin K. Outcome reporting in industry-sponsored trials of gabapentin for off-label use. *N Engl J Med* 2009;361:1963-71.

31 Ross JS, Madigan D, Hill KP, Egilman DS, Wang Y, Krumholz HM. Pooled analysis of rofecoxib placebo-controlled clinical trial data: lessons for postmarket pharmaceutical safety surveillance. *Arch Intern Med* 2009;169:1976-85.

32 Psaty BM, Kronmal RA. Reporting mortality findings in trials of rofecoxib for Alzheimer disease or cognitive impairment: A case study based on documents from rofecoxib litigation. *JAMA* 2008;299:1813-7.

33 Bero L. Implications of the tobacco industry documents for public health and policy. *Annu Rev Public Health* 2003;24:267-88.

34 Dundar Y, Dodd S, Dickson R, Walley T, Haycox A, Williamson PR. Comparison of conference abstracts and presentations with full-text articles in the health technology assessments of rapidly evolving technologies. *Health Technol Assess* 2006;10(5).

35 Higgins JPT, Green S, eds. 6.2.2.4 Conference abstracts or proceedings. In: *Cochrane handbook for systematic reviews of interventions* . Version 5.1.0. Cochrane Collaboration, 2011. Available from www.cochrane-handbook.org.

36 Hartling L, Bond K, Vandermeer B, Seida J, Dryden DM, Rowe BH. Applying the risk of bias tool in a systematic review of combination long-acting beta-agonists and inhaled corticosteroids for persistent asthma. *PLoS One* 2011;6:e17242.

37 Krumholz HM, Ross JS. A model for dissemination and independent analysis of industry data. *JAMA* 2011;306:1593-4.

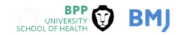

Interpreting diagnostic accuracy studies for patient care

Susan Mallett, medical statistician[1], Steve Halligan, professor of radiology[2], Matthew Thompson, GP, senior clinical scientist, codirector of Oxford Centre for Monitoring and Diagnosis[1], Gary S Collins, senior medical statistician[3], Douglas G Altman, professor of statistics in medicine[3]

[1]University of Oxford, Department of Primary Care Health Sciences, Oxford OX2 6GG, UK

[2]University College London, Centre for Medical Imaging, London, NW1 2BU, UK.

[3]University of Oxford, Centre for Statistics in Medicine, Oxford, OX2 6UD

Correspondence to: S Mallett susan.mallett@phc.ox.ac.uk

Cite this as: BMJ 2012;344:e3999

DOI: 10.1136/bmj.e3999

http://www.bmj.com/content/345/bmj.e3999

Studies of tests that aim to diagnose clinical conditions that are directly applicable to daily practice should present test results that are directly interpretable in terms of individual patients— for example, the number of true positive and false positive diagnoses. We do not examine measures used for early experimental (exploratory) studies, in which diagnostic thresholds have not been established.

Results obtained from a diagnostic test accuracy study are expressed by comparison with a reference standard of the "true" disease status for each patient. Thus, once a clinically relevant diagnostic threshold has been established, patients' results can be categorised by the test as true positive (TP), false positive (FP), true negative (TN), and false negative (FN) (fig 1).

Diagnostic accuracy can be presented at a specific threshold by using paired results such as sensitivity and specificity, or alternatively positive predictive value (PPV) and negative predictive value (NPV) (see fig 1). Other methods summarise accuracy over a range of different test thresholds—for example, the area under the receiver operator curve (ROC AUC, see fig 1).

Despite the simplicity of the 2×2 structure, the presentation and interpretation of tests and comparisons between them are not straightforward. Graphical presentation can be highly informative, in particular an ROC plot, which is a plot of sensitivity against 1−specificity (or false positive rate). Figure 2 shows an ROC plot of test accuracy of a single test at different thresholds. ROC plots are also used within studies to compare different tests, to compare different groups of patients, and to investigate variability between different test observers (readers). ROC plots are useful in systematic reviews to present results from multiple studies.

Several concepts need to be considered carefully in the interpretation of data from a diagnostic accuracy study:

- How does accuracy change with different diagnostic thresholds?
- If paired outcomes (such as sensitivity and specificity) are compared for different scenarios, they often change

ABSTRACT

A diagnostic test accuracy study provides evidence on how well a test correctly identifies or rules out disease and informs subsequent decisions about treatment for clinicians, their patients, and healthcare providers. The authors highlight several different ways in which data from diagnostic test accuracy studies can be presented and interpreted, and discuss their advantages and disadvantages.

in opposite directions. For example, sensitivity is of higher in one test and specificity higher in the ot Which is more important?

- What are the clinical consequences of a missed (fa negative) diagnosis or a false positive diagnosis? these risks be presented together—for example, a relative benefit?
- What is the best way to include disease prevalence in summary of clinical benefit?
- Are results presented in terms of what happens individual patients, which are often the easiest clinicians (and their patients) to understand?[1]

Reporting test accuracy at different thresholds

Presenting results at a single threshold

When a test has only a single threshold or cutpoint value instance, positive or negative for disease, such as a biops results are naturally presented in pairs, usually sensitiv and specificity, or PPV and NPV (see fig 1). Although (and NPV equivalently) allow easy comprehension of probability that a patient with a positive test result has disease, when tests are compared in the same patient is not straightforward to use these measures because calculation of confidence intervals is complex.[2]

Tests that yield results on a continuous scale requ specification of a test threshold to define positive a negative results. Changing the threshold alters proportion of false positive and false negative diagnos Figure 2 shows how the sensitivity of CA19-9 for diagno of pancreatic cancer increases as the threshold value lowered from 1000 to 15 U/ml, while specificity decrease

Presenting results at multiple thresholds

For many diagnostic tests, however, there are multi potential thresholds at which different clinical decisio could be made, often reflecting diagnostic uncertain For example, the mammographic BI-RADS classification breast screening has six categories: 0=additional imag evaluation required; 1=negative; 2=benign findin 3=probably benign finding; 4=suspicious abnormality; a 5=highly suggestive of malignancy.[3]

SUMMARY BOX

- Diagnostic test accuracy studies should present data in a way that is comprehensible and relevant to clinicians, their patients, and healthcare providers when making clinical management decisions
- The most relevant and applicable presentation of diagnostic test results allows inclusion of four key components: interpretation in terms of patients; clinically relevant values for test threshold(s); realistic disease prevalence; and clinically relevant relative gains and losses in terms of patients (that is, true positive and false positive diagnoses)
- Presenting diagnostic accuracy as paired measures, such as sensitivity and specificity, or as net benefit summaries with component paired measures, allows inclusion of these four components whereas using the area under the ROC curve as a diagnostic performance measure does not

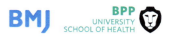

Diagnostic accuracy measures
Diagnostic test results are expressed in comparison with reference standard diagnosis of disease

	Reference standard test	
	Disease positive	Disease negative
Test positive	True positive (TP)	False positive (FP)
Test negative	False negative (FN)	True negative (TN)

Paired diagnostic measures at specific thresholds (such as sensitivity and specificity)
Sensitivity is the proportion of patients (or test results) with disease correctly diagnosed using a specific threshold to define a positive test result

$$Sensitivity = \frac{TP}{(TP + FN)}$$

Specificity is the proportion of patients (or test results) without disease correctly diagnosed

$$Specificity = \frac{TN}{(TN + FP)}$$

Other paired diagnostic measures include: positive predictive value (PPV) and negative predictive value (NPV) or positive (LR+) and negative (LR−) likelihood ratios

Single diagnostic measure across multiple test thresholds: for example, area under the ROC curve (ROC AUC)

ROC AUC is the area under the ROC curve of sensitivity v 1−specificity

The ROC AUC for each test corresponds to the probability that of two randomly chosen people, one with and one without disease, the diagnostic test will rank the person with disease with a higher suspicion of disease than the one without disease. For example, an ROC AUC of 0.7 means that of two randomly chosen people, there is a 70% chance (equivalent to a 0.7 probability) that the person with disease will be ranked with higher suspicion than the person without disease. An alternative interpretation of the ROC AUC is the average sensitivity given that all values of specificity are equally likely[27]
Other single diagnostic measures used include the H-measure[21] (where misclassification costs can be fixed) and the diagnostic odds ratio (DOR)[28]

Fig 1 Diagnostic accuracy measures

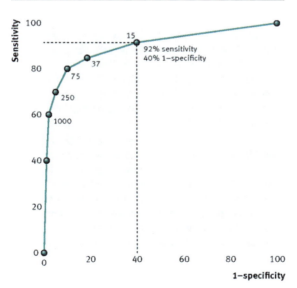

Fig 2 ROC plot of test accuracy at different thresholds. Data from systematic review of CA19-9.[29] Threshold values are shown in U/mL. At 15 U/mL, test accuracy is 92% sensitivity and 60% specificity (1−specificity=40%)

For many diagnostic tests there is no consensus regarding the clinically optimal threshold that separates a positive from a negative result as it is difficult to agree at which threshold it is acceptable to risk missing disease. With measures such as sensitivity and specificity, diagnostic accuracy can be reported for each test threshold relevant to

the management of patients. Even then, it is important to understand that not all thresholds are equally important. For the diagnosis of breast cancer with the BI-RADS scale, the threshold between "highly suggestive of malignancy" and "suspicious abnormality" is clearly more clinically important to a patient and her doctor than the threshold between "benign" and "probably benign."

Presenting a performance measure combined across thresholds
Alternatively, diagnostic accuracy can be summarised by combining accuracy across a range of thresholds with a measure such as ROC AUC (fig 1).[4] This, however, can be a disadvantage if thresholds that are clinically relevant are combined with those that are clinically nonsensical.[5] Clinically, information is needed on how a test performs in patients at a clinically relevant threshold rather than a summary of how the test might perform across all possible thresholds.

Are false positive and false negative diagnoses equally important?
No diagnostic test is perfect and almost all tests will sometimes miss disease or indicate disease in normal patients (see FN and FP, respectively, in fig 1). False negative and false positive diagnoses, however, are rarely equally important. Missing a life threatening disease will probably be regarded by a patient (and his or her doctor) as much more important than a false positive diagnosis in a healthy patient. For example, a study of attitudes and knowledge of mammography for screening for breast cancer found that 63% of women thought that 500 or more women receiving false positive results was reasonable for each life saved.[6]

The relative importance of a false negative versus a false positive diagnosis (also called relative misclassification cost) varies according to where the test fits in the patient pathway and who is making the assessment. For example, funders or commissioners of healthcare might have a different perspective from patients or clinicians as additional false positive diagnoses will increase costs. The relative importance of additional false negative versus additional false positive diagnoses is particularly important in decisions about which of two tests is "better"—which is more important, an increase in sensitivity or an increase in specificity? To evaluate which test is better, performance needs to incorporate clinical costs.

Presenting diagnostic accuracy for patients
For diagnostic accuracy studies to usefully inform clinical practice, their results should be related to decisions regarding management of patients. Presentation in terms of individual patients is often best,[1] and formats such as animations with smiley faces have been successful.[7]

Interpretation in terms of patients is straightforward and direct for paired measures such as sensitivity and specificity, PPV and NPV, or positive and negative likelihood ratios. Sensitivity and specificity provide test accuracy in terms of patients in a population, although interpretation for an individual patient with unknown disease status is less obvious. PPV and NPV are useful to understand the probability that a patient with a given positive or negative test result has a diagnosis of disease. Positive and negative likelihood ratios are useful to understand the role of a test result in changing a clinician's estimate of the probability of disease in a patient. These paired measures can be combined into a single measure (for example, "net benefit" measure; see below), which is also easily understood, particularly when it is reported with the component paired measures.

By contrast, interpretation of a single numerical value of the ROC AUC is problematic because the summary across all thresholds is difficult to reconcile with a specific threshold for the individual patient. Also ROC AUC is hard to interpret in practice, as it is the probability that randomly selected pairs of patients, one with and one without disease, would be ordered correctly for probability of disease (see fig 1). However, patients do not walk into the clinician's room in pairs,[8] and patients want their results and diagnosis, rather than the order of their results compared with another patient.

Comparing the performance of two diagnostic tests

Three main approaches can be used to compare the diagnostic accuracy of two tests that differ depending on whether a specific test threshold is used or performance is averaged across multiple thresholds. They also vary in whether they can be interpreted in terms of patients and whether they can incorporate clinical context, such as relative weightings of false negative and false positive diagnoses and also disease prevalence. Ideally, diagnostic tests should be compared within the same patients or, if this is not practical, on randomised groups from the same population of patients. This ensures that differences in observed test results are because of the tests rather than differences in characteristics of patients or study methods.

Paired measures at specific thresholds

The first method compares two tests according to differences in paired measures such as sensitivity and specificity. For example, of two biomarker tests for pancreatic cancer, CA 19-9 with 83% sensitivity and 81% specificity can be compared with CA 242 with a sensitivity of 74% and specificity of 91%: CA 19-9 has 9% higher sensitivity, but 10% lower specificity.[9] The clinical context of these differences in sensitivity and specificity would be enhanced by using clinically relevant disease prevalence to report the difference in the actual number of patients with true and false positive diagnoses. For a given increase in sensitivity, if the prevalence of disease is twice as high, then the number of patients who receive a true positive diagnosis is doubled. Nevertheless, paired measures are transparent enough for healthcare providers or patients to incorporate their own relevant contextual information.

Summary measure at specific thresholds: net benefit methods

In the second approach, a single overall measure of diagnostic performance can be presented by using net benefit or net utility methods, calculated from test performance at a specific clinically relevant threshold.[10] [11] [12] [13] [14] [15] [16] [17] Several of these measures are based directly on the difference in sensitivity and specificity between the two tests being compared at one[10] [13] [18] or more than one clinical threshold.[16] [19] A single overall measure of diagnostic performance is often preferred for simplicity when guiding healthcare spending or regulatory approval decisions. These methods directly incorporate the contextual information regarding prevalence and relative importance of false negative and false positive diagnoses.

The weighted comparison (WC) net benefit measure[13] method weights differences in sensitivity and specificity between two tests by the relative clinical costs and disease prevalence (see box). With the previous example of CA 19-9 and CA 242, the net benefit is positive (weighted comparison=0.07) if CA 19-9 is used instead of CA 242, a disease prevalence of 33%, and a 10-fold higher relative weighting of true positive diagnoses over false positive diagnoses (box). To aid interpretation, the weighted comparison can be converted to a net benefit equivalent to 23 more true positive test results per 1000 patients based on actual values of 30 more patients receiving a true positive result and 66 more patients receiving a false positive diagnosis.

Single measure averaged across multiple thresholds

A third approach calculates a single overall measure of diagnostic accuracy but averaged across multiple test thresholds—for example, ROC AUC[20] (fig 1) and the new H-measure.[21] We illustrate ROC AUC with two tumour markers measured on the same patients[9]; CA 19-9 seems to be the superior test as it has an AUC of 0.86, which is greater than 0.70 for CA 125 (fig 3).

Problems with ROC AUC for diagnostic performance

The use and interpretation of ROC AUC as a measure of diagnostic performance highlights several advantages[6] and disadvantages.[4] [22] Somewhat surprisingly, ROC AUC remains the recommended measure of effectiveness for some evaluations of devices submitted to the US Food and Drug Administration, for example in imaging and computer aided detection.[23]

AUC or partial AUC?

The standard ROC AUC averages across all possible thresholds. Not all test thresholds, however, are clinically relevant.[5] For many tests, thresholds offering high sensitivity (such as greater than 80%) are not clinically useful because specificity is too low (see fig 3a and b); patients with false positive results would overwhelm diagnostic services. One way to deal with this is to calculate a partial ROC AUC (pAUC) thus restricting comparisons to sensible thresholds.[24] For example, by excluding sensitivity above 80%, the partial ROC AUC is 0.27 for CA 125 and 0.15 for CA 19-9, suggesting that CA 125 is the superior test (see fig 3c and d). It could also be argued that a sensitivity of less than 70% is unlikely to be clinically useful (too little disease would be detected). pAUC therefore restricted to the range between 70% and 80% sensitivity produces values of 0.12 for CA 125 and 0.11 for CA 19-9, suggesting the tests are equally effective (fig 3e and f).

This example illustrates a dilemma in ROC AUC interpretation. Should the AUC be calculated across all test thresholds (including those that are clinically illogical[5] [25]) or should a pAUC be calculated, restricted to clinically sensible thresholds? If a partial AUC approach is taken, as illustrated in figure 3, even small changes in the choice of threshold can affect which test has the greater AUC and is classified as superior.[26]

Extrapolation beyond available data

The choice between standard AUC or pAUC needs particular consideration when available data are restricted to a small region of the ROC plot space. To calculate a standard AUC the ROC curve must be extrapolated beyond the available data, so that the whole AUC encompassing 0% to 100% sensitivity can be calculated. This is a key issue in systematic reviews in which data from included studies are often limited to a small region of ROC space.

Moreover, the extrapolated region of the curve dominates the AUC as it includes the right hand side of the plot, which dominates the ROC AUC. This region lacks clinical importance because it is based on thresholds where over-

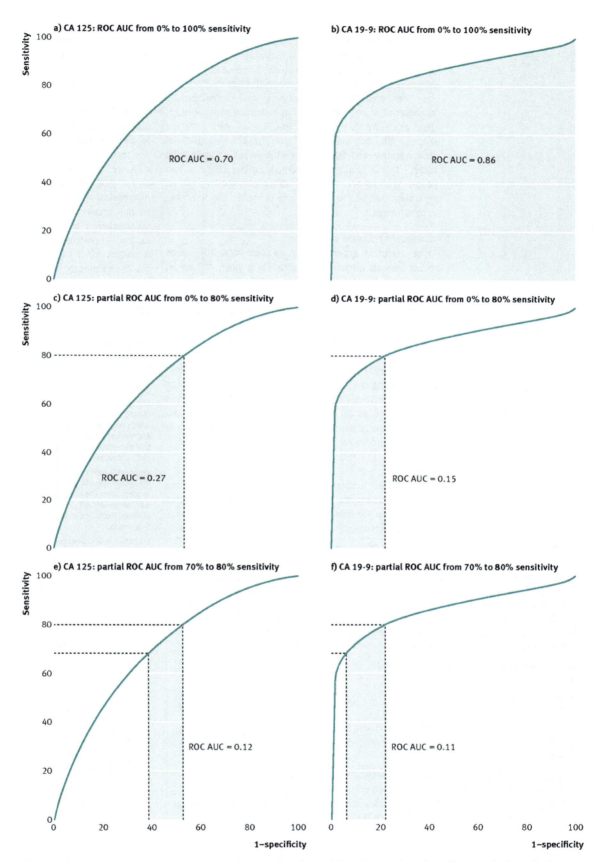

Fig 3 Use of ROC AUC to compare two tests: CA 19-9 and CA 125. Shaded areas indicate ROC AUC for regions of interest. Blood samples from 51 control patients with pancreatitis and 90 patients with pancreatic cancer were analysed for CA 125 and CA 19-9[31]

half the patients receive false positive results. The poor utility of the full AUC has been noted in breast screening, where high specificity is important to avoid large numbers of false positive results leading to unnecessary biopsies in a population with a low prevalence.[25]

Incorporating relative misclassification costs

ROC AUC does not allow incorporation of the relative clinical consequences of false negative and false positive diagnoses. It is often believed that ROC AUC uses equally balanced misclassification costs for these diagnoses, but this applies only at one point on the ROC curve, where the gradient equals one. In reality, the misclassification costs for false negative and false positive diagnoses vary along the ROC curve and are dictated by its shape[14] and therefore do not relate to any clinically meaningful information. This has been described as nonsensical and fundamentally incoherent.[27] If ROC AUC is used as a performance measure, then when we compare two ROC curves with different shapes, different balances of misclassification costs of false negative and false positive diagnoses underlie each curve.[21] This is analogous to comparing the height of two people by using only the numerical output from two rulers, regardless that one ruler measures in inches and the other in centimetres.[27]

Incorporating disease prevalence

To be useful as a performance measure, ROC AUC needs to use realistic disease prevalence. For a given ROC curve, the calculated AUC is the same regardless of the underlying prevalence of the study data, given the same disease severity. When ROC AUC is used to compare two tests, this is sometimes wrongly perceived as evaluation at 50% prevalence. As with misclassification costs, unless the ROC curve corresponds to a straight line, it is not possible to fix a single disease prevalence with ROC AUC, as the gradient changes along the curve. To our knowledge this issue has not been previously highlighted. This is problematic when ROC AUC is used to compare tests because the absolute benefit of the difference in sensitivity and specificity is clearly dependent on disease prevalence.

Summary

Diagnostic test accuracy studies need to provide evidence in a comprehensible and intuitive format that facilitates choice of test for clinicians, their patients, and healthcare providers. Results should be reported in the context of clinical management decisions made at clinically sens and important thresholds, preferably in terms of patie For comparisons of tests, differences in true positive false positive diagnoses should be reported, and i important that any overall measures of diagnostic accur should incorporate relative misclassification costs account for the fact that false negative and false posi diagnoses are rarely clinically equivalent. Measures n to be interpreted at a disease prevalence that refl the real clinical situation. Analyses based on net ben measures achieve these aims. In contrast, methods ba on ROC AUC often incorporate thresholds that are clinic nonsensical, do not account for disease prevalence, cannot account for the differing clinical implications false negative and false positive diagnoses. We theref caution researchers against solely reporting ROC measures when summarising diagnostic performance, caution healthcare providers against using ROC AUC al to inform decisions regarding diagnostic performance. recommend that diagnostic accuracy is presented by us paired measures with clinical context or using net ben measures with their associated paired measures.

Contributors: SM initiated the manuscript based on discussions o the topic with the other authors, who all contributed to manuscri drafting. SM is guarantor.

Funding: This work was funded by UK Department of Health via a National Institute for Health Research (NIHR) programme grant (RP-PG-0407-10338) and Cancer Research UK programme grant (C5529). A proportion of this work was undertaken at UCLH/UCL, which receives a proportion of funding from the NIHR Comprehen Biomedical Research Centre funding scheme. The views expressed this publication are those of the authors and not necessarily thos the UK Department of Health.

Competing interests: All authors have completed the ICMJE uniform disclosure form at www.icmje.org/coi_disclosure.pdf (available on request from the corresponding author) and declare that Medicsig plc (Hammersmith, London) funded research relating to computer assisted detection that precipitated some of the views expressed this article.

Provenance and peer review: Not commissioned; peer reviewed.

NET BENEFIT METHODS TO MEASURE DIAGNOSTIC PERFORMANCE

Net benefit measures can provide an overall impact across changes in paired measures. For example, the weighted comparison (WC) measure[13] is an index weighting the difference in sensitivity and difference in specificity of two tests, taking into account the relative clinical cost (misclassification costs) of a false positive compared with a false negative diagnosis and disease prevalence. We note that the WC measure is similar to the net reclassification index (NRI),[14] if the latter is adapted to account for disease prevalence and relative misclassification costs.

WC=⊘sensitivity+[(1−prevalence/prevalence)×relative cost (FP/TP)×⊘specificity]

What do weighted comparison values mean?

- Positive WC values indicate a net benefit
- Zero WC values show no net benefit
- Negative WC values show a net loss
- 95% confidence intervals and thresholds for clinical benefit are used to indicate significance of results. To aid interpretation, WC can be converted into an equivalent increase in true positive patients per 1000.

Example calculating WC for two biomarker tests of pancreatic cancer

Comparing two tumour marker tests for diagnosis of pancreatic cancer, CA 19-9 with 83% sensitivity and 81% specificity to CA 242 with 74% sensitivity and 91% specificity,[9] the difference in sensitivity (⊘sensitivity) is 9% (equivalent to 0.09) and the difference in specificity (⊘specificity) is −10% (or −0.10). So in a population with estimated disease prevalence of 33%, and a 10-fold higher relative weighting for true positive diagnoses compared with false positive diagnoses, the WC is obtained as:

WC=0.09−(2×0.1×0.10)=0.07As WC is positive there is an increased net benefit favouring CA 19-9. To aid interpretation, WC can be converted into an equivalent increase in true positive patients per 1000, if all the benefit was focused into TP patients by calculating WC×prevalence×1000.

A WC of 0.07 converts to a benefit equivalent to 23 more true positive patient results per 1000 patients, based on actual values of 30 more patients receiving a true positive result and 66 more patients receiving a FP diagnosis, at prevalence and relative weighting as specified.

Other single diagnostic measures include: other net effect measures[10] [11] [12] [15] [16] [17] [30] and net reclassification index.[14]

1   Gigerenzer G, Gaissmaier W, Kurz-Mileke E, Schwartz LM, Woloshin Helping doctors and patients make sense of health statistics. Psyc Sci Public Interest 2008;8:53-96.
2   Leisenring W, Alonzo T, Pepe MS. Comparisons of predictive values of binary medical diagnostic tests for paired designs. Biometrics 2000;56:345-51.
3   D'Orsi CJ, Mendelson EB, Ikeda DM. Breast imaging reporting and system: ACR BI-RADS-Breast Imaging Atlas. In: D'Orsi CJ, Bassett LW Berg WA, eds. BI-RADS: Mammography. American College of Radiol 2003.
4   Wagner RF, Metz CE, Campbell G. Assessment of medical imaging systems and computer aids: a tutorial review. Acad Radiol 2007;14:723-48.
5   Greenland S. The need for reorientation toward cost-effective prediction: comments on 'Evaluating the added predictive ability a new marker: from area under the ROC curve to reclassification a beyond' by Pencina MJ, et al. Statistics in Medicine (doi:10.1002/ sim.2929). Stat Med 2008;27:199-206.
6   Schwartz LM, Woloshin S, Sox HC, Fischhoff B, Welch HG. US wome attitudes to false-positive mammography results and detection of ductal carcinoma in situ: cross-sectional survey. West J Med 2000;173:307-12.
7   Speigelhalter D. Understanding uncertainty. 2011. http:// understandinguncertainty.org/view/animations.
8   Pepe MS, Feng Z, Gu JW. Comments on 'Evaluating the added predictive ability of a new marker: from area under the ROC curve to reclassification and beyond' by Pencina MJ, et al. Statistics in Medicine (doi:10.1002/sim.2929). Stat Med 2008;27:173-81.
9   Haglund C, Lundin J, Kuusela P, Roberts PJ. CA 242, a new tumour marker for pancreatic cancer: a comparison with CA 19-9, CA 50 ar CEA. Br J Cancer 1994;70:487-92.
10   Adams NM, Hand DJ. Comparing classifers when the misallocation costs are uncertain. Pattern Recognition 1999;32:1139-47.
11   DeNeef P, Kent DL. Using treatment-tradeoff preferences to select diagnostic strategies: linking the ROC curve to threshold analysis. Med Decis Making 1993;13:126-32.
12   Lusted LB. Decision-making studies in patient management. N Eng Med 1971;284:416-24.
13   Moons KG, Stijnen T, Michel BC, Buller HR, Van Es GA, Grobbee DE, al. Application of treatment thresholds to diagnostic-test evaluatio

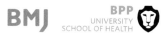

an alternative to the comparison of areas under receiver operating characteristic curves. *Med Decis Making* 1997;17:447-54.

14   Pencina MJ, D'Agostino RB Sr, D'Agostino RB Jr, Vasan RS. Evaluating the added predictive ability of a new marker: from area under the ROC curve to reclassification and beyond. *Stat Med* 2008;27:157-72.

15   Vergouwe Y, Steyerberg EW, Eijkemans MJ, Habbema JD. Validity of prognostic models: when is a model clinically useful? *Semin Urol Oncol* 2002;20:96-107.

16   Vickers AJ, Elkin EB. Decision curve analysis: a novel method for evaluating prediction models. *Med Decis Making* 2006;26:565-74.

17   Wagner RF, Beam CA, Beiden SV. Reader variability in mammography and its implications for expected utility over the population of readers and cases. *Med Decis Making* 2004;24:561-72.

18   Peirce CS. The numerical measure of the success of predictions. *Science* 1884;IV:453-4.

19   Vickers AJ, Cronin AM, Elkin EB, Gonen M. Extensions to decision curve analysis, a novel method for evaluating diagnostic tests, prediction models and molecular markers. *BMC Med Inform Decis Mak* 2008;8:53.

20   Wagner RF, Beiden SV, Campbell G, Metz CE, Sacks WM. Assessment of medical imaging and computer-assist systems: lessons from recent experience. *Acad Radiol* 2002;9:1264-77.

21   Hand DJ. Evaluating diagnostic tests: the area under the ROC curve and the balance of errors. *Stat Med* 2010;29:1502-10.

22   Hilden J. The area under the ROC curve and its competitors. *Med Decis Making* 1991;11:95-101.

23   Gallas BD, Chan HP, D'Orsi CJ, Dodd LE, Giger ML, Gur D,et al. Evaluating imaging and computer-aided detection and diagnosis devices at the FDA. *Acad Radiol* 2012;19:463-77.

24   Thompson ML, Zucchini W. On the statistical analysis of ROC curves. *Stat Med* 1989;8:1277-90.

25   Baker SG. The central role of receiver operating characteristic (ROC) curves in evaluating tests for the early detection of cancer. *J Natl Cancer Inst* 2003;95:511-5.

26   Walter SD. The partial area under the summary ROC curve. *Stat Med* 2005;24:2025-40.

27   Hand D.J. Measuring classifier performance: a coherent alternative to the area under the ROC curve. *Mach Learn* 2009;77:103-23.

28   Glas AS, Lijmer JG, Prins MH, Bonsel GJ, Bossuyt PM. The diagnostic odds ratio: a single indicator of test performance. *J Clin Epidemiol* 2003;56:1129-35.

29   Niederau C, Grendell JH. Diagnosis of pancreatic carcinoma. Imaging techniques and tumor markers. *Pancreas* 1992;7:66-86.

30   Bandos AI, Rockette HE, Gur D. Incorporating utility-weights when comparing two diagnostic systems: a preliminary assessment. *Acad Radiol* 2005;12:1293-300.

31   Wieand S, Gail MH, James BR, James KL. A family of nonparametric statistics for comparing diagnostic markers with paired or unpaired data. *Biometrika* 1989;76:585-92.

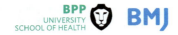

Demystifying trial networks and network meta-analysis

Edward J Mills, associate professor[1][2], Kristian Thorlund, associate professor[2][3], John P A Ioannidis, professor[2][4]

[1]Faculty of Health Sciences, University of Ottawa, 35 University Drive, Ottawa, ON, Canada, K1N 6N5

[2]Stanford Prevention Research Center, Department of Medicine, Stanford University School of Humanities and Sciences, Stanford, CA, USA

[3]Department of Clinical Epidemiology and Biostatistics, McMaster University, Hamilton, ON, Canada

[4]Department of Health Research and Policy, Stanford University School of Medicine, and Department of Statistics, Stanford University School of Humanities and Sciences, Stanford, CA, USA

Correspondence to: E J Mills Edward. mills@uottawa.ca.

Cite this as: BMJ 2013;346:f2914

DOI: 10.1136/bmj.f2914

http://www.bmj.com/content/346/bmj.f2914

Introduction

When multiple interventions have been used and compared for the same disease and outcomes, network meta-analysis (also commonly referred to as a multiple treatment comparison meta-analysis or mixed treatment meta-analysis) offers a set of methods to visualize and interpret the wider picture of the evidence and to understand the relative merits of these multiple interventions.[1] Network meta-analysis has advantages over conventional pairwise meta-analysis, as the technique borrows strength from indirect evidence to gain certainty about all treatment comparisons and allows for estimation of comparative effects that have not been investigated head to head in randomized clinical trials.[2] For this reason, network meta-analysis is quickly gaining popularity among clinicians, guideline developers, and health technology agencies as new evidence on new interventions continues to surface and needs to be placed in the context of all available evidence for appraisals.[3] For example, over the past two decades more than 20 randomized clinical trials have investigated the long term (>12 months) effects of several variants of warfarin and aspirin as well as other drug treatments for the prevention of stroke in patients with non-rheumatic atrial fibrillation. This accumulation of evidence on multiple treatments has resulted in a network of interventions and comparisons (such as the resulting treatment network, fig 1) that constitutes the randomized evidence between all interventions. In contrast to conventional pairwise meta-analysis, network meta-analysis can provide estimates of relative efficacy between all interventions, even though some have never been compared head to head. For many comparisons, the network meta-analysis may yield more reliable and definitive results than would a pairwise meta-analysis.

In spite of the increasing popularity and widespread use network meta-analysis, certain methodological and interpretational aspects are poorly understood. The strength of evidence and risk of bias for each of the involved comparisons and in the treatment network as a whole[4]; the analytical challenges, tools, and opportunities in

ABSTRACT

Networks of randomized clinical trials can be evaluated in the context of a network meta-analysis, a procedure that permits inferences into the comparative effectiveness of interventions that may or may not have been evaluated directly against each other. This approach is quickly gaining popularity among clinicians and guideline decision makers. However, certain methodological aspects are poorly understood. Here, we explain the geometry of a network, statistical and conceptual heterogeneity and incoherence, and challenges in the application and interpretation of data synthesis. These concepts are essential to make sense of a network meta-analysis.

detecting and exploring heterogeneity within and between comparisons[5]; and the interpretation of widely used statistical models and effect measures are all matters that deserve further elucidation to ensure high quality synthesis of evidence in the setting of multiple interventions.[6] Here we aim to demystify these key challenges and opportunities offered by trial networks and network meta-analyses in the context of a working example of interventions for preventing stroke in patients with non-rheumatic atrial fibrillation.[7]

Part 1: network geometry

A key element to understanding a treatment network is the evaluation of its geometry.[8] That is, which of the considered treatments (nodes) have been compared head to head in randomized controlled trials, which of the considered treatments are connected indirectly through one or more "common comparators," and what is the level of evidence informing each comparison. By examining the connections between interventions in a graphical way, as in figure 1, a reader can determine how strong the evidence is for the treatment network as a whole and for the individual comparisons, whether specific comparisons are over-represented or under-represented, and whether the network is well connected. The better connected a network is, the more reliable the estimates it provides will be. Figure 1 illustrates an example of the geometry in a treatment network. This figure includes 34 randomized pairwise comparisons, of which warfarin (n=20), aspirin (n=16), and placebo (n=12) have the most links.[7] The most common comparison (n=7 trials) is between warfarin and aspirin (the two most commonly tested treatments), and the network includes four comparisons of each of them against placebo, the third most common comparator. Overall, 45 possible pairwise comparisons can be made between the nine treatments. Of these, 16 comparisons are informed directly by head to head evidence, but six of the direct connections have only one trial. Thus several of the comparisons that have not been directly studied are informed by indirect evidence from only two trials. Nodes in a network that are not well connected, such as indobufen and ximelagatran in this example, should be interpreted with caution. The diversity and strength of a network are determined by the number

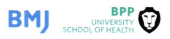

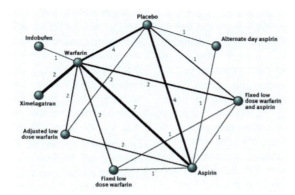

Fig 1 Network geometry of well connected network of randomized controlled trials (RCTs) evaluating stroke prevention among populations with atrial fibrillation. Circles represent the drug as a node in the network; lines represent direct comparisons using RCTs; thickness of lines represents the number of RCTs included in each comparison, also represented by the numbers

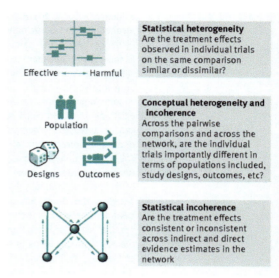

Statistical heterogeneity
Are the treatment effects observed in individual trials on the same comparison similar or dissimilar?

Conceptual heterogeneity and incoherence
Across the pairwise comparisons and across the network, are the individual trials importantly different in terms of populations included, study designs, outcomes, etc?

Statistical incoherence
Are the treatment effects consistent or inconsistent across indirect and direct evidence estimates in the network

Fig 2 Common considerations of heterogeneity and inconsistency in a network

of different interventions and comparisons of interventions that are available, how represented they are in the network, and how much evidence they carry. Severe imbalance in terms of the amount of evidence for each intervention may affect the power and reliability of the overall analysis,[9] [10] as inferences may be driven largely from the evidence on one or a few treatments and comparisons. The treatment network in figure 1 is a fairly diverse treatment network. Some comparisons are informed by several randomized clinical trials (both directly and indirectly), whereas other comparisons are only sparsely informed (either by direct or indirect evidence).

Many pairwise meta-analyses are insufficiently powered,[11] and similar problems may extend to network analyses.[10] Evidence that is procured by small trials tends to be susceptible to greater bias (for example, more prominent publication and selective reporting biases),[12] and small trials may spuriously show larger treatment effects.[13] Combination of such biased results may yield unreliable estimates in a network. Because networks include evidence from both direct and indirect comparisons, power may be better than in simple pairwise meta-analyses that include only direct evidence.[10] However, the uncertainty of the results in networks with limited evidence should not be underestimated and may extend beyond what the results of any traditional data synthesis might show.[10]

Peculiar co-occurrence patterns suggesting comparator preference biases may also exist—for example, most new drugs may be compared against an established inactive comparator (placebo) or a straw man intervention (one that is known to be a poor choice) rather than against the standard of care, or some head to head comparisons may be avoided. For example, in some fields (such as treatment of partial epilepsy with second generation antiepileptic drugs[8] or biologic drugs for rheumatoid arthritis[14]) placebo controlled trials are almost exclusively performed. This may result to some extent from guidance and requirements by regulatory agencies or may represent the choice of industry sponsors. However, sometimes, the lack of specific direct head to head comparisons may simply be due to a lack of attention to important comparisons that need to be looked at in the future. For example, for most neglected tropical diseases, few or no head to head comparisons have been done between the two or three treatments that are recommended by guidelines as main treatments.[15] Trials in this field are rarely sponsored by the industry. This lack

of specific informative comparisons cannot be documented robustly unless the whole network of comparisons is visualized. Identification of missing evidence on specific essential comparisons can guide the performance of the most informative trials in the future research agenda.

Part 2: heterogeneity and incoherence

Network meta-analysis offers a unique opportunity to probe whether homogeneity or heterogeneity exists in the results of different trials in each of the pairwise comparisons that it includes and whether coherence or incoherence is present in the results of different trials that inform indirect comparisons versus the respective available evidence from direct comparisons.

Figure 2 summarizes the concepts of statistical and conceptual heterogeneity and incoherence. Statistical and conceptual aspects overlap but are not identical. Statistical heterogeneity is tested by tests such as Cochran's Q and quantified by metrics such as I^2.[16] In the example of interventions for stroke prevention, none of the pairwise comparisons has evidence of statistically significant heterogeneity ($P>0.10$ for all on the Q test). However, only three of the available pairwise comparisons were informed by more than two trials, so very little power was available to detect any potential heterogeneity statistically. Although not statistically proven, heterogeneity can still be present and can often be checked conceptually. Conceptual heterogeneity refers to differences in methods, study design, study populations, settings, definitions and measurements of outcome, follow-up, co-interventions, or other features that make trials different. In network meta-analysis, such differences are gauged in the same way as they are in conventional pairwise meta-analysis. However, in network meta-analysis one needs to keep in mind that multiple comparisons are involved. For this reason, conceptual heterogeneity should be assessed both within each comparison and between all comparisons. In our example, conceptual heterogeneity between trials is apparent as a varying proportion of the included patient populations had a history of stroke or transient ischemic attack (ranging from 0% to 100%), despite the fact that all trials were designed to evaluate comparative treatment effects in non-rheumatic atrial fibrillation.[7]

Conceptual heterogeneity across comparisons can result in discrepant results from direct evidence and indirect evidence.[17] Such discrepancies are termed incoherence. Incoherence can occur only when both direct and indirect evidence inform the same comparison. For example, for a comparison between treatments A and B, randomized clinical trials must have compared A and B head to head and both interventions with some common comparator, C. This is commonly referred to as a closed loop. Incoherence can exist only in closed loops, and the presence of incoherence can be assessed by comparing the point estimates of the direct and indirect evidence informing the same comparison. This can be done informally by gauging the overlap of the uncertainty intervals accompanying the point estimates, or it can be done formally by statistically testing differences between the direct and indirect point estimate. In the treatment network for stroke prevention interventions, one nominal signal of incoherence was detected for one among the 10 treatment loops in the network—the treatment loop of placebo, aspirin, and adjusted low dose warfarin. Here, the indirect evidence suggested a large, clearly statistically significant reduction in incidence rate ratio (per 1000 person years) of atrial fibrillation events in favor of adjusted low dose warfarin versus aspirin (0.23, 95% confidence interval 0.10 to 0.63), whereas the direct evidence suggested no effect (incidence rate ratio of adjusted low dose warfarin versus aspirin 0.97, 0.47 to 1.94).

Considering the apparent conceptual heterogeneity in connection with the limited power to detect statistical heterogeneity and incoherence, results of the network meta-analysis should therefore be interpreted with caution. At the same time, we should caution that statistical testing for both heterogeneity and incoherence is subject not only to type II error (lack of power to detect heterogeneity/incoherence, when evidence is sparse) but also to type I error (false positive detection of heterogeneity/incoherence, especially when many tests are performed, as in a very complex network). This means that in most network meta-analyses, finding no nominally significant signals for incoherence does not fully exclude its presence, and finding an occasional nominally significant signal of incoherence may sometimes be a false positive. Neither statistical diagnostics nor conceptual reasoning alone is perfect, but their careful combined consideration may be optimal.[18]

When clear conceptual heterogeneity and incoherence are seen, one has to consider whether synthesizing the results across trials in a network meta-analysis is justifiable. When statistical heterogeneity or incoherence is detected, one needs to think carefully about whether clear conceptual explanations for it exist or whether the signal is a chance finding. Furthermore, if one cannot conceptu[ally] explain the detected statistical heterogeneity, incoheren[ce] or both, one has to decide whether combining the dat[a in] the same network makes sense and whether the res[ults] should be interpreted with extra caution. Random eff[ect] meta-analysis models can accommodate unexplai[ned] heterogeneity for the available pairwise comparisons [and] often also make the incoherence signals less prominent[.]

We should also acknowledge that we lack solid evide[nce] on whether the results of network meta-analyses w[ith] evidence of heterogeneity and incoherence have [less] reliability, and thus have poorer ability to predict the res[ults] of a future trial on a comparison of interest. In the larg[est] evaluation to examine the coherence between direct [and] indirect evidence, Song et al evaluated 112 independent [meta-]networks (including 1552 trials with 478 775 patients) t[hat] allowed a test for difference between direct and indi[rect] evidence.[19] Incoherence was statistically significant in [16] cases (14% of tests), yet the direction of treatment eff[ect] only differed in two cases.

Part 3: data synthesis

Different models exist for synthesizing data in netw[ork] meta-analyses.[20] The choice of model may affect the amo[unt] of confidence one can statistically put in the point estima[tes] produced. The two most widely used models in netw[ork] meta-analysis (and conventional pairwise meta-analy[sis) are the fixed effect model and the random effects model. [The] fixed effect model assumes that no (or a negligible amo[unt] of) heterogeneity exists. This assumption is recogni[zed] to be typically unrealistic. When heterogeneity exists [and] the fixed effect model is applied, uncertainty inter[vals] (for example, 95% credible intervals) become artifici[ally] narrow. For this reason, the random effects model, wh[ich] does assume and account for unexplained heterogene[ity,] is typically preferred. Returning to our stroke preven[tion] example, some evidence of both statistical and concept[ual] heterogeneity was identified. For this reason, the rand[om] effects model seems the appropriate choice.

One of the most appealing but misunderstood eleme[nts] of network meta-analysis is the reporting of probabili[ties] of which treatment is the best, followed by next best, a[nd] so on. Various methods of displaying probabilities [are] used.[21] A risk exists that one may incorrectly emphas[ize] the probabilities as being clinically useful when [the] treatment effects are, in fact, not different from the [rest] beyond chance.[4] Probabilities can be fragile when [the] network is sparse. The ranking of treatments may cha[nge] drastically when a new trial is introduced into a netwo[rk.] For that reason, authors should place less emphasis on [the] probabilities of a network meta-analysis output and grea[ter] emphasis on the treatment effects and their uncertainty.

Returning to our example from figure 1, table 1 sho[ws] the rate ratio with credible intervals (that is, Bayes[ian] confidence intervals) of each treatment compared w[ith] placebo and the associated probability that each treatm[ent] is best. Only for four of the eight active treatments [do] we have sufficient confidence that they are better th[an] placebo. Nevertheless, when we calculated the probabilit[ies] of being best, alternate day aspirin was associated with [the] largest probability (66%) of being the best treatment, ev[en] though it is one of the four treatments for which we ha[ve] no confidence that its effect is any better than placebo. T[his] discrepancy occurs because alternate day aspirin yields [the] largest point estimate for treatment effect (compared w[ith] placebo), and most of the probability mass for its treatm[ent] effect is centered around small rate ratios.

Table Treatment effect estimates from example network

Network comparator treatments	Rate ratio (95% credible interval)	Treatment	Probability of being best treatment (%)
—	—	Placebo	0
Adjusted standard dose warfarin v placebo	0.37 (0.26 to 0.53)	Adjusted standard dose warfarin	3
Adjusted low dose warfarin v placebo	0.32 (0.18 to 0.56)	Adjusted low dose warfarin	16
Fixed low dose warfarin v placebo	0.76 (0.30 to 1.76)	Fixed low dose warfarin	1
Aspirin v placebo	0.62 (0.43 to 0.86)	Aspirin	0
Fixed low dose warfarin and aspirin v placebo	0.98 (0.60 to 1.67)	Fixed low dose warfarin and aspirin	0
Ximelagatran v placebo	0.35 (0.19 to 0.65)	Ximelagatran	11
Alternate day aspirin v placebo	0.17 (0.01 to 1.15)	Alternate day aspirin	66
Indobufen v placebo	0.46 (0.19 to 1.14)	Indobufen	5

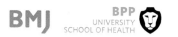

Summary

Treatment networks and network meta-analysis of randomized trials offer an exceptional opportunity to understand how much evidence is available for each treatment and treatment comparison, where and why more evidence is needed, where and why heterogeneity and incoherence exist, and what the best available treatments are, as well as the uncertainty surrounding such assessments. As network meta-analyses become more popular and influential, familiarity with these opportunities and challenges will be necessary for providing transparent and reliable evidence synthesis.

We are grateful to Steve Kanters for statistical assistance and Georgia Salanti for providing available trial level data.

Contributors: All authors conceived, drafted, and revised the paper for important critiques and approved the final submission.

Competing interests: All authors have completed the ICMJE uniform disclosure form at www.icmje.org/coi_disclosure.pdf (available on request from the corresponding author) and declare: no support from any organization for the submitted work; no financial relationships with any organizations that might have an interest in the submitted work in the previous three years; no other relationships or activities that could appear to have influenced the submitted work.

Provenance and peer review: Not commissioned; externally peer reviewed.

1 Lu G, Ades AE. Combination of direct and indirect evidence in mixed treatment comparisons. *Stat Med* 2004;23:3105-24.
2 Caldwell DM, Ades AE, Higgins JP. Simultaneous comparison of multiple treatments: combining direct and indirect evidence. *BMJ* 2005;331:897-900.
3 Sutton A, Ades AE, Cooper N, Abrams K. Use of indirect and mixed treatment comparisons for technology assessment. *Pharmacoeconomics* 2008;26:753-67.
4 Mills EJ, Ioannidis JP, Thorlund K, Schunemann HJ, Puhan MA, Guyatt GH. How to use an article reporting a multiple treatment comparison meta-analysis. *JAMA* 2012;308:1246-53.
5 Jansen JP, Fleurence R, Devine B, Itzler R, Barrett A, Hawkins N, et al. Interpreting indirect treatment comparisons and network meta-analysis for health-care decision making: report of the ISPOR Task Force on Indirect Treatment Comparisons Good Research Practices: part 1. *Value Health* 2011;14:417-28.
6 Coleman CI, Phung OJ, Cappelleri JC, Baker WL, Kluger J, White CM, et al. Use of mixed treatment comparisons in systematic reviews. [Publisher?], 2012.
7 Cooper NJ, Sutton AJ, Lu G, Khunti K. Mixed comparison of stroke prevention treatments in individuals with nonrheumatic atrial fibrillation. *Arch Intern Med* 2006;166:1269-75.
8 Salanti G, Kavvoura FK, Ioannidis JP. Exploring the geometry of treatment networks. *Ann Intern Med* 2008;148:544-53.
9 Mills EJ, Ghement I, O'Regan C, Thorlund K. Estimating the power of indirect comparisons: a simulation study. *PLoS One* 2011;6:e16237.
10 Thorlund K, Mills EJ. Sample size and power considerations in network meta-analysis. *Syst Rev* 2012;1:41.
11 Guyatt GH, Oxman AD, Kunz R, Brozek J, Alonso-Coello P, Rind D, et al. GRADE guidelines 6: rating the quality of evidence—imprecision. *J Clin Epidemiol* 2011;64:1283-93.
12 Ioannidis JP, Cappelleri JC, Lau J. Issues in comparisons between meta-analyses and large trials. *JAMA* 1998;279:1089-93.
13 Pereira TV, Horwitz RI, Ioannidis JP. Empirical evaluation of very large treatment effects of medical interventions. *JAMA* 2012;308:1676-84.
14 Thorlund K, Druyts E, Avina-Zubieta JA, Wu P, Mills EJ. Why the findings of published multiple treatment comparison meta-analyses of biologic treatments for rheumatoid arthritis are different: an overview of recurrent methodological shortcomings. *Ann Rheum Dis* 2012; published online 20 Oct.
15 Kappagoda S, Ioannidis JP. Neglected tropical diseases: survey and geometry of randomised evidence. *BMJ* 2012;345:e6512.
16 Higgins JP, Thompson SG, Deeks JJ, Altman DG. Measuring inconsistency in meta-analyses. *BMJ* 2003;327:557-60.
17 Ioannidis JP. Integration of evidence from multiple meta-analyses: a primer on umbrella reviews, treatment networks and multiple treatments meta-analyses. *CMAJ* 2009;181:488-93.
18 Pereira TV, Patsopoulos NA, Salanti G, Ioannidis JP. Critical interpretation of Cochran's Q test depends on power and prior assumptions about heterogeneity. *Research Synthesis Methods* 2010;1:12.
19 Song F, Xiong T, Parekh-Bhurke S, Loke YK, Sutton AJ, Eastwood AJ, et al. Inconsistency between direct and indirect comparisons of competing interventions: meta-epidemiological study. *BMJ* 2011;343:d4909.
20 Dias S, Welton N, Sutton A, Ades AE. NICE DSU technical support document 1: introduction to evidence synthesis for decision-making. 2012. www.nicedsu.org.uk/TSD1Introduction.final.08.05.12.pdf.
21 Salanti G, Ades AE, Ioannidis JP. Graphical methods and numerical summaries for presenting results from multiple-treatment meta-analysis: an overview and tutorial. *J Clin Epidemiol* 2011;64:163-71.

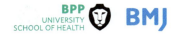

Interpreting and reporting clinical trials with results of borderline significance

Allan Hackshaw, deputy director[1], Amy Kirkwood, statistician[1]

[1]Cancer Research UK and UCL Cancer Trials Centre, University College London, London W1T 4TJ

Correspondence to: Allan Hackshaw ah@ctc.ucl.ac.uk

Cite this as: BMJ 2011;343:d3340

DOI: 10.1136/bmj.d3340

http://www.bmj.com/content/343/bmj.d3340

The quality of randomised clinical trials and how they are reported have improved over time, with clearer guidelines on conduct and statistical analysis.[1] Clinical trials often take several years, but interpreting the results at the end is arguably the most important activity because it influences whether a new intervention is recommended or not. Although researchers have become more familiar with medical statistics, the interpretation and reporting of results of borderline significance remains a problem. We examine the problem and recommend some solutions.

What is the problem?

New interventions used to be compared with minimal or no treatment, so researchers were looking for and finding large treatment effects. Clear recommendations were made because the P values were usually small (eg, P<0.001). However, modern interventions are usually compared with the existing standard treatment, so that the effects are often expected to be smaller than before, and it is no longer as easy to get small P values. The cut-off used to indicate a real effect is widely taken as P=0.05 (called statistically significant). The problem is that although P=0.05 is an arbitrary figure, many researchers still adhere strictly to it when making conclusions about an intervention, and often use it as the sole basis for this. Researchers and journals sometimes conclude that there is no effect.

The P=0.05 cut-off was first proposed by R A Fisher in 1925 as being low enough to make decisions, and over time has become widely adopted. However, examining interventions with P values just above 0.05 is difficult, especially if the trial is unique. It is incorrect to regard, for example, a relative risk of 0.75 with a 95% confidence interval of 0.57 to 0.99 and P=0.048 as clear evidence of an effect, but the same point estimate with a 95% confidence interval of 0.55 to 1.03 and P=0.07 as showing no effect, simply because one P value is just below 0.05 and the other just above. Although the issue has been raised before,[2][3] it still occurs in practice.

P values are an error rate (like the false positive rate in medical screening). In the same way that a small P value does not guarantee that there is a real effect, a P value just above 0.05 does not mean no effect. If P=0.049, we expect to claim that a new intervention is beneficial, when it really is not, almost 5% of the time, but the intervention would probably still be recommended. The size of a P value depends on two factors: the magnitude of the treatment

ABSTRACT

Borderline significance in the primary end point of trials does not necessarily mean that the intervention is not effective. Researchers and journals need to be more consistent in how they report these results

effect (relative risk, hazard ratio, mean difference, etc) and the size of the standard error (which is influenced by the study size, and either the number of events or standard deviation, depending on the type of outcome measure used). Very small P values (the easiest to interpret) arise when the effect size is large and the standard error is small. Borderline P values can occur when there is a clinically meaningful treatment effect but a large or moderate standard error—often because of an insufficient number of participants or events (the trial is referred to as being underpowered). This is perhaps the most common cause of borderline results. Borderline P values can also occur when the treatment effect is smaller than expected, which with hindsight would have a required a larger trial to produce a value <0.05, so again the study is underpowered.

Using confidence intervals

Confidence intervals are usually more informative than the P value when borderline results are found, as the following example shows. The EICESS-92 phase III trial aimed to determine whether adding etoposide to standard ifosfamide chemotherapy would improve event-free survival in Ewing's sarcoma.[4] Powered to detect a hazard ratio of 0.60 (40% relative risk reduction), the target sample size was 400 patients (492 were recruited). The observed hazard ratio was 0.83 (95% confidence interval 0.65 to 1.05, P=0.12). Because P>0.05 it would normally be concluded that there is insufficient evidence for an effect, even though the 17% risk reduction is clinically important, but smaller than the 40% expected. Most researchers and journal reviewers understand that the true effect is likely to lie somewhere in the confidence interval range, hence the possibility of being 1.0—that is, no effect. However, there is a common misconception that the true effect lies anywhere within the range with equal likelihood. It is more likely to be around the estimated hazard ratio (0.83, the best estimate of the true effect) than at either extremes of the confidence interval. Thus, although the upper limit (1.05) is just above the no effect value, there is only a 6% chance that it exceeds 1.0 (figure). There is a 50% chance that the true hazard ratio is between 0.77 and 0.90, or 75% chance that it is between 0.71 and 0.95; therefore a treatment benefit is likely. The authors concluded that "the addition of etoposide seemed to be beneficial." This is appropriate wording because it is the only randomised study to evaluate adding etoposide to an ifosfamide regimen in this patient group, and the disorder is uncommon (it took 6.5 years to recruit 492 patients). Even 7.5 years after recruitment had ended the number of events (n=266) still did not allow the primary end point to have P<0.05. To conclude insufficient evidence or, worse still

SUMMARY POINTS

- Many researchers still adhere too strictly to the arbitrary P cut-off value of 0.05 when interpreting clinical trial results
- A P value that is just above 0.05 does not mean that there is no effect
- Confidence intervals are a better indicator of the likelihood of an effect and its size
- The true effect of an intervention is more likely to lie around the middle of a confidence interval (that is, the point estimate) than at either end
- Authors and journals should be more consistent in how they report primary trial end points of borderline significance

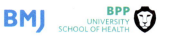

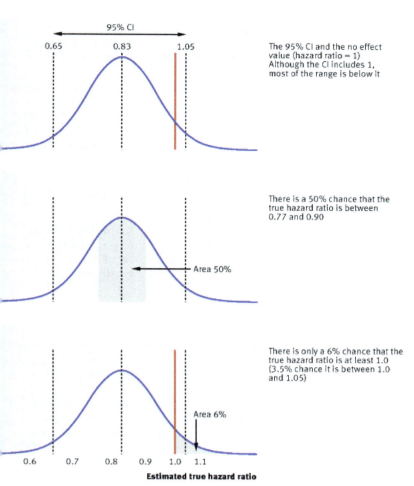

The 95% CI and the no effect value (hazard ratio = 1) Although the CI includes 1, most of the range is below it

There is a 50% chance that the true hazard ratio is between 0.77 and 0.90

Area 50%

There is only a 6% chance that the true hazard ratio is at least 1.0 (3.5% chance it is between 1.0 and 1.05)

Area 6%

Interpreting the results of a trial with hazard ratio 0.83 and 95% confidence interval 0.65 to 1.05. The vertical broken lines indicate the point estimate and the lower and upper confidence limits; the solid line is the no effect value

no effect, would have been incorrect and a useful result from a unique trial would be missed. Although the target sample size was exceeded, the observed treatment effect was smaller than originally expected, hence the lack of statistical significance.

Inconsistency in language in clinical trial reports

We examined the *BMJ, Lancet, JAMA, New England Journal of Medicine, Journal of the National Cancer Institute,* and the *Journal of Clinical Oncology* to see how the results or conclusions of randomised phase III trials published in 2009 were described in the abstract (which most readers focus on). Out of 287 studies, 24 (1 in 12) were considered to have borderline results when the direction of the primary end point indicated a treatment benefit, with P value between 0.05 and 0.10 or a lower or upper 95% confidence limit close to the no effect value (that is, 1 for risk or hazard ratios and 0 for risk or mean differences). The table gives examples and a full list is available on bmj.com.[5-28] There is a general inconsistency in the language used. The intention here is not to alter the published conclusions, but only to be aware of the differences in how they were reported.

Among 10 article abstracts that concluded or gave the impression of no effect for the primary end point, seven had P values of 0.11 to 0.17 with hazard or odds ratios ranging from 0.85 to 0.90 and upper 95% confidence limits of 1.02 to 1.07, and one had a mean difference of 0.06×10^3 (95% confidence interval −0.002 to 0.13×10^3) with a P value of 0.06.[5] These results suggest that there is probably some effect, but perhaps not clinically worthwhile. However, a seemingly large

effect was found in two trials with P=0.06 and upper 95% confidence limits just above the no effect value (table). One had a mean difference in scores of −27.8 units[7] and the other a relative risk of 0.66,[11] so there probably is a real benefit on the primary end point in both cases.

Eleven articles concluded that there was a suggestion of an effect, usually with moderate to large treatment effects, and P values 0.06 to 0.10 (often 0.06 or 0.07). However, in one trial the effect seemed relatively small (hazard ratio=0.93, 95% confidence interval 0.84 to 1.02, P=0.13[19]). All of these articles seemed to base their conclusions not just on the P value but on other end points or adjusted results. In two trials, the achieved sample size was much lower than the target because of poor accrual, but both found large treatment effects (hazard ratios 0.67 and 0.69), which would probably have been significant if there had been more patients.[22 24]

Three articles concluded an effect with some confidence. The treatment effects were variable, and P values ranged between 0.06 and 0.1. Again, authors sometimes drew attention to other significant end points but the language in relation to the main outcome measure could have been less strong in some cases.

Although seven of the 24 studies were large (≥2000 participants), this did not guarantee clear results for the primary end point. The overall conclusions of several studies were often supported by results for other end points or from other trials, and the possibility of an effect was discussed outside the abstract. However, it is inconsistent that, for example, two trials with similar effect sizes (risk ratios of 0.66 and 0.67) and P values (0.06 and 0.07) came to different conclusions (no effect [11] and suggestion of an effect[24]), and two trials with a smaller effect size (hazard ratio 0.84) but similar or larger P value (0.06 or 0.13) indicated a possible effect (table).[19 25] It is also useful to consider borderline confidence intervals and P values when a trial intervention unexpectedly suggests harm in relation to the primary end point. Authors might be more inclined to make firmer conclusions in this situation than if an intervention shows evidence of benefit. However, we found two examples where there were more events in the intervention group but the authors concluded only that there was no benefit. In a randomised trial of 635 patients with type 2 diabetes and diabetic retinopathy, the primary end point was developing clinically important macular oedema[29]; the hazard ratio for calcium dobesilate versus placebo was 1.32 (0.96 to 1.81, P=0.08), but the conclusion in the abstract stated only that calcium dobesilate did not reduce the risk of developing macular oedema. Similarly, in a trial of 486 head and neck cancer patients comparing gefitinib (250 or 500 mg) with methotrexate,[30] the hazard ratios for mortality were 1.22 (P=0.12) and 1.12 (P=0.39) for 250 and 500 mg, respectively. The conclusion reported in the abstract stated that "neither gefitinib 250 nor 500 mg/day improved overall survival," though the pooled hazard ratio would be 1.17 (95% confidence interval 0.98 to 1.39).

Possible solutions

The problem of borderline results could be avoided by designing trials with small or moderate effect sizes. However, this is often not feasible because large sample sizes are usually required, which is particularly challenging in uncommon disorders. But even with careful trial design and good prior evidence, the observed treatment effect can be noticeably lower than that expected, thus producing P values that are just above 0.05 (as in the Ewing's sarcoma

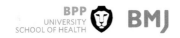

Table Examples of randomised phase III trials with borderline positive results but different author interpretations

Trial and author interpretation	Interventions and patient group (No of participants)	Primary end point	Main result (95% CI), P value	Conclusion in abstract
No effect on primary end point was concluded or implied				
Bakitas et al[7]	Nurse led psycho-educational intervention v usual care for palliative care in patients with advanced cancer (n=322)	Symptom intensity (quality of life and resource use were other end points)	Mean difference in score −27.8 (−57.2 to 1.6), P=0.06	"Those receiving nurse-led ... haintervention ... had higher scores for quality of life and mood but did not have improvements in symptom intensity scores"
Murphy et al[11]	Tailored care plan v usual care in patients with coronary heart disease (n=903)	Patients with systolic blood pressure >140 mm Hg at 18 months (hospital admission was another end point)	Odds ratio 0.66 (0.43 to 1.01), P=0.06	"Admissions to hospital we significantly reduced...but n other clinical benefits were shown"
Lefebvre et al[12]	Alternating v sequential chemotherapy and radiotherapy in patients with resectable advanced squamous cell carcinoma of the larynx or hypopharynx (n=450)	Survival with a functional larynx	Hazard ratio 0.93 (0.84 to 1.02), P=0.15	"Larynx preservation, progression-free interval, a overall survival were simila in both arms"
Suggestion of effect on primary end point				
O'Connor et al[19]	Aerobic exercise training plus usual care v usual care alone, in patients with chronic heart failure (n=2331)	All cause mortality or hospital admission	Hazard ratio 0.93 (0.84 to 1.02), P=0.13	"Exercise training resulted nonsignificant reductions in the primary endpoint"
Stahl et al[24]	Pre-surgical chemoradiotherapy v chemotherapy in patients with locally advanced cancer of the oesophagogastric junction (n=126, target was 576)	Overall survival	Hazard ratio 0.67 (0.41 to 1.07), P=0.07	"Although...statistical significance was not achieved, results point to a survival advantage for preoperative chemoradiotherapy"
Albain et al[25]	Cyclophosphamide, doxorubicin, and fluorouracil (CAF) followed by tamoxifen v CAF given concurrently with tamoxifen, in breast cancer(n=1116)	Disease-free survival	Hazard ratio 0.84 (0.70 to 1.01),P=0.06	"The adjusted HRs favoured CAF-T [sequential] over CAFT [concurrent] but did not reach significance for disease-free survival"
Clear effect on primary end point				
Jabre et al[27]	Ketamine versus etomidate among patients requiring sedation for emergency intubation (n=469)	Organ system function, determined from the maximum sequential organ failure assessment	Mean difference −0.7 (−1.4 to 0.0), P=0.056	"Our results show that ketamine is a safe and valuable alternative to etomidate"
Peterson et al[28]	Personalised telephone counselling using cognitive behavioural skills v no intervention to encourage smoking cessation in adolescents (n=2151)	6 months abstinence from smoking	Absolute risk difference 4.0% (−0.2% to 8.1%), P=0.06	"Personalized motivational interviewing ... is effective in increasing teen smoking cessatior"

trial above). A possible solution is to use a validated and established surrogate marker as the primary (or co-primary) end point—for example, progression-free survival instead of overall survival in some cancer trials, or cholesterol for some prevention trials in cardiovascular disease. There should be more events if a surrogate marker is used, and this will increase the chance of the result being statistically significant. However, researchers need to be aware that finding significant results for a true end point (such as survival) will be difficult because such studies are smaller. Furthermore, borderline results could still be found with any end point.

Meta-analysis can also be a solution, but only if there are two or more trials to combine. This was indeed the case for one of the articles we found,[15] where the hazard ratio

for one trial was 0.86, 95% confidence interval 0.72 to (P=0.08), but the pooled effect from three trials was o 0.75 to 0.98 (P=0.02). However, there are many instan when the trial is the only one and will not be repea usually because of greater interest in newer intervention because limitations of sample size or rarity of the disor make it unfeasible to repeat the trial. Unique trials m become more common because international clinical t registers now allow researchers to check if similar stud are in progress elsewhere. Although it is generally g practice to have at least two trials of the same interven (with consistent results) before recommending it routine use, researchers might be less inclined to cond a replicate trial or be less likely to receive a grant fr funding organisations.

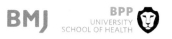

Recommendations

The figure shows why a confidence interval is a better way of interpreting data when borderline results are found. Importantly, it shows that even when P>0.05, there is a higher likelihood that the true effect lies around the point estimate from the trial, rather than at the ends of the confidence interval, so a treatment effect should not be readily dismissed if it seems clinically meaningful.

Borderline results cannot be used as strong evidence either for or against an intervention. If a clinically important effect is observed with a P value just above 0.05 (or an upper or lower confidence limit close to the no effect value), it is incorrect to conclude no effect and not consider further what is likely to be an effective intervention, especially for uncommon disorders or trials that took many years to complete. Researchers should examine other end points to look for consistency and other evidence (for example, cohort studies, dose-response relations, or similar types of treatments that show a clear effect). Importantly, they should state that there is evidence for the primary end point but use moderate words such as "suggestion," "seems," or "indication" that need to be accepted consistently by journals. If the treatment effect is lower than expected, the clinical implications could be specifically discussed. The aim is to avoid giving the reader the impression that an intervention is completely ineffective, when it is likely to be effective. Similarly, researchers of trials with results of borderline significance should not give the impression that the evidence is conclusive. The same principles apply to other areas of research such as examining risk factors for and causes of disorders or early death.

We thank Nicholas Wald for his helpful comments.

Competing interest: All authors have completed the ICJME unified disclosure form at www.icmje.org/coi_disclosure.pdf (available on request from the corresponding author) and declare no support from any organisation for the submitted work; no financial relationships with any organisation that might have an interest in the submitted work in the previous three years; and no other relationships or activities that could appear to have influenced the submitted work.

Contributors: AH had the original idea, AK reviewed the journals to identify clinical trial reports that had borderline results, and both authors reviewed the articles, wrote the paper, and approved the final version. AH is the guarantor.

1   Moher D, Schulz KF, Altman DG. THE CONSORT statement: revised recommendations for improving the quality of reports of parallel-group randomized trials. *Ann Intern Med* 2001;134:657-62.
2   Altman DG, Bland JM. Absence of evidence is not evidence of absence. *BMJ* 1995;311:485.
3   Alderson P. Absence of evidence is not evidence of absence. *BMJ* 2004;328:476.
4   Paulussen M, Craft AW, Lewis I, Hackshaw A, Weston C, Douglas C, et al. The European Intergroup Cooperative Ewing's Sarcoma Study Group. EICESS-92—results of two randomised trials of the European Intergroup Cooperative Ewing's Sarcoma Study. *J Clin Oncol* 2008;26:4385-93.
5   ASTRAL Investigators. Revascularization versus medical therapy for renal-artery stenosis. *N Engl J Med* 2009;361:1953-61.
6   Azzopardi DV, Strohm B, Edwards AD, Dyet L, Halliday HL, Juszczak E, et al. Moderate hypothermia to treat perinatal asphyxial encephalopathy. *N Engl J Med* 2009;361:1349-58.
7   Bakitas M, Lyons KD, Hegel MT, Balan S, Brokaw FC, Seville J, et al. Effects of a palliative care intervention on clinical outcomes in patients with advanced cancer: the Project ENABLE II randomized controlled trial. *JAMA* 2009;302:741-9.
8   Bhatt DL, Lincoff AM, Gibson CM, Stone GW, McNulty S, Montalescot G, et al. Intravenous platelet blockade with cangrelor during PCI. *N Engl J Med* 2009;361:2330-41.
9   Duckworth W, Abraira C, Moritz T, Reda D, Emanuele N, Reaven PD, et al. Glucose control and vascular complications in veterans with type 2 diabetes. *N Engl J Med* 2009;360:129-39.
10   Mehta SR, Granger CB, Boden WE, Steg PG, Bassand JP, Faxon DP, et al. Early versus delayed invasive intervention in acute coronary syndromes. *N Engl J Med* 2009;360:2165-75.
11   Murphy AW, Cupples ME, Smith SM, Byrne M, Byrne MC, Newell J, et al. Effect of tailored practice and patient care plans on secondary prevention of heart disease in general practice: cluster randomised controlled trial. *BMJ* 2009;339:b4220.
12   Lefebvre JL, Rolland F, Tesselaar M, Bardet E, Leemans CR, Geoffrois L, et al. Phase 3 randomized trial on larynx preservation comparing sequential vs alternating chemotherapy and radiotherapy. *J Natl Cancer Inst* 2009;101:142-52.
13   Löwenberg B, Ossenkoppele GJ, van Putten W, Schouten HC, Graux C, Ferrant A, et al. High-dose daunorubicin in older patients with acute myeloid leukemia. *N Engl J Med* 2009;361:1235-48.
14   Van Cutsem E, Labianca R, Bodoky G, Barone C, Aranda E, Nordlinger B, et al. Randomised phase III trial comparing biweekly infusional fluorouracil/leucovorin alone or with irinotecan in the adjuvant treatment of stage III colon cancer: PETACC-3. *J Clin Oncol* 2009;27:3117-25.
15   Cunningham D, Chau I, Stocken DD, Valle JW, Smith D, Steward W, et al. Phase III randomized comparison of gemcitabine versus gemcitabine plus capecitabine in patients with advanced pancreatic cancer. *J Clin Oncol* 2009;27:5513-8.
16   Fidias PM, Dakhil SR, Lyss AP, Loesch DM, Waterhouse DM, Bromund JL, et al. Phase III study of immediate compared with delayed docetaxel after front-line therapy with gemcitabine plus carboplatin in advanced non-small-cell lung cancer. *J Clin Oncol* 2009;27:591-8.
17   Grau MV, Sandler RS, McKeown-Eyssen G, Bresalier RS, Haile RW, Barry EL, et al. Nonsteroidal anti-inflammatory drug use after 3 years of aspirin use and colorectal adenoma risk: observational follow-up of a randomized study. *J Natl Cancer Inst* 2009;101:267-76.
18   Hess G, Herbrecht R, Romaguera J, Verhoef G, Crump M, Gisselbrecht C, et al. Phase III study to evaluate temsirolimus compared with investigator's choice therapy for the treatment of relapsed or refractory mantle cell lymphoma. *J Clin Oncol* 2009;27:3822-9.
19   O'Connor CM, Whellan DJ, Lee KL, Keteyian SJ, Cooper LS, Ellis SJ, et al. Efficacy and safety of exercise training in patients with chronic heart failure: HF-ACTION randomized controlled trial. *JAMA* 2009;301:1439-50.
20   Plint AC, Johnson DW, Patel H, Wiebe N, Correll R, Brant R, et al. Epinephrine and dexamethasone in children with bronchiolitis. *N Engl J Med* 2009;360:2079-89.
21   Rerks-Ngarm S, Pitisuttithum P, Nitayaphan S, Kaewkungwal J, Chiu J, Paris R, et al. Vaccination with ALVAC and AIDSVAX to prevent HIV-1 infection in Thailand. *N Engl J Med* 2009;361:2209-20.
22   Roh MS, Colangelo LH, O'Connell MJ, Yothers G, Deutsch M, Allegra CJ, et al. Preoperative multimodality therapy improves disease-free survival in patients with carcinoma of the rectum: NSABP R-03. *J Clin Oncol* 2009;27:5124-30.
23   Soligard T, Myklebust G, Steffen K, Holme I, Silvers H, Bizzini M, et al. Comprehensive warm-up programme to prevent injuries in young female footballers: cluster randomised controlled trial. *BMJ* 2008;337:a2469.
24   Stahl M, Walz MK, Stuschke M, Lehmann N, Meyer HJ, Riera-Knorrenschild J, et al. Phase III comparison of preoperative chemotherapy compared with chemoradiotherapy in patients with locally advanced adenocarcinoma of the esophagogastric junction. *J Clin Oncol* 2009;27:851-6.
25   Albain KS, Barlow WE, Ravdin PM, Farrar WB, Burton GV, Ketchel SJ, et al. Adjuvant chemotherapy and timing of tamoxifen in postmenopausal patients with endocrine-responsive, node-positive breast cancer: a phase 3, open-label, randomised controlled trial. *Lancet* 2009;374:2055-63.
26   Gomes MF, Faiz MA, Gyapong JO, Warsame M, Agbenyega T, Babiker A, et al. Pre-referral rectal artesunate to prevent death and disability in severe malaria: a placebo-controlled trial. *Lancet* 2009;373:557-66.
27   Jabre P, Combes X, Lapostolle F, Dhaouadi M, Ricard-Hibon A, Vivien B, et al. Etomidate versus ketamine for rapid sequence intubation in acutely ill patients: a multicentre randomised controlled trial. *Lancet* 2009;374:293-300.
28   Peterson AV Jr, Kealey KA, Mann SL, Marek PM, Ludman EJ, Liu J, et al. Group-randomized trial of a proactive, personalized telephone counseling intervention for adolescent smoking cessation. *J Natl Cancer Inst* 2009;101:1378-92.
29   Haritoglou C, Gerss J, Saverland C, Kampik A, Ulbig MW, et al. Effect of calcium dobesilate on occurrence of diabetic macular oedema (CALDIRET study): randomised, double-blind, placebo-controlled, multicentre trial. *Lancet* 2009;373:1364-71.
30   Stewart JSW, Cohen EEW, Licitra L, Van Herpen CML, Khorprasert C, Soulieres D, et al. Phase III study of gefitinib compared with intravenous methotrexate for recurrent squamous cell carcinoma of the head and neck. *J Clin Oncol* 2009;27:1864-71.

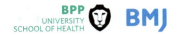

Statistics Notes: Missing outcomes in randomised trials

Andrew J Vickers, attending research methodologist[1],
Douglas G Altman, professor of statistics in medicine[2]

[1]Department of Epidemiology and Biostatistics, Memorial Sloan-Kettering Cancer Center, New York, NY 10065, USA

[2]Centre for Statistics in Medicine, University of Oxford, Oxford OX2 6UD, UK

Correspondence to: A Vickers vickersa@mskcc.org

Cite this as: BMJ 2013;346:f3438

DOI: 10.1136/bmj.f3438

http://www.bmj.com/content/346/bmj.f3438

In most randomised trials, some patients fail to provide data for study endpoints.[1] We have previously described the analysis of a trial of acupuncture versus sham acupuncture for the treatment of shoulder pain.[2] All 52 randomised patients provided baseline data on pain and range of motion, but only 45 returned for follow-up testing. The statistical question is how to handle those seven patients with missing data. The most straightforward approach is simply to ignore the seven patients and do what is known as an "available case analysis" (often confusingly known as "complete case analysis"). As not all randomised patients are included in the analysis, this leads to reduced statistical power.[1]

A method that attempts to include all randomised patients is "last observation carried forward," in which the last measurement obtained from the patient is used for all data points that were subsequently missed. This method is attractive because it is simple, but it has little else to recommend it. Substituting a missing data point with a value is known as "imputation,"[1] and the data analyst needs a clear rationale for the type of imputation used. That a patient's responses would remain the same after drop-out is generally implausible. This is most obvious in chronic degenerative diseases. For instance, cognitive function scores decrease over time in dementia, so last observation carried forward gives overoptimistic scores for patients who drop out (figure). If a treatment was associated with toxicity, and this led to earlier drop-out than in the control group, the method would give results biased in favour of the experimental arm.[3] By contrast, shoulder pain generally gets better over time, either because treatment is effective or because of the placebo effect and regression to the mean.[4] In the randomised trial, patients in the control group improved by a mean of 9.8 points out of 100 from baseli[...] to post-treatment follow-up, whereas patients who receiv[...] acupuncture improved by 21.5 points. So assuming th[...] patients lost to follow-up experienced precisely zero chan[...] in pain scores makes little sense. Last observation carri[...] forward may also underestimate the standard deviati[...] of the endpoint, especially in cases in which the la[...] observation is the baseline, leading to confidence interva[...] that are too narrow.

A more sophisticated approach to missing data is kno[...] as multiple imputation, which uses a regression model [...] predict missing values.[5] In randomised trials, the stronge[...] predictors of future outcome are often the scores provid[...] by the patient so far, but other variables can be included. [...] avoid underestimating the width of the confidence interv[...] multiple imputation involves a form of random samplin[...] For a given patient with a missing outcome, regression [...] used to predict the mean value of the missing outcome [...] similar patients and also the variability around the mea[...] a value is then selected at random from this distributio[...] The results from several imputations (hence "multiple[...] are combined using a method known as "Rubin's rules."[...] Multiple imputation is widely believed to be the preferr[...] approach to missing data, not just for randomised trial[...] It is computationally complex, however, and needs [...] be implemented by special software, such as the "ic[...] command in Stata (see www.multiple-imputation.com).

The table shows the results of the shoulder pain stu[...] analysed by each method. The estimates for available ca[...] and multiple imputation do not differ much, althou[...] multiple imputation has a slightly narrower confiden[...] interval. Last observation carried forward appears to [...] biased—it underestimates the effects of acupuncture—a[...] gives a confidence interval that is too narrow.

Multiple imputation works best when good predicto[...] of outcome are available. In the shoulder pain examp[...] baseline score was only moderately correlated wi[...] follow-up score (r≈0.4). Had outcome been assesse[...] halfway through treatment, this measure would have be[...] more highly correlated with post-treatment score, marked[...] improving the properties of the multiple imputation.

Multiple imputation has several important strengths, b[...] it does not adjust for the sort of bias created if patien[...] were less likely to return for follow-up if they were in a lot [...] pain; this is an inherent limitation to missing data analys[...] We cannot know whether patients' pain levels affe[...] the chance that they will complete a pain questionnai[...] because, obviously enough, we do not have the pain scor[...] of non-respondents.

Sometimes simple common sense is more important th[...] complex statistics. In the shoulder pain trial, three of t[...] seven drop-outs were in the acupuncture group and fo[...] were controls, so it seems implausible that their omissi[...] had materially affected the results of the trial. If drop-o[...] rates were very different between the two arms of a tri[...]

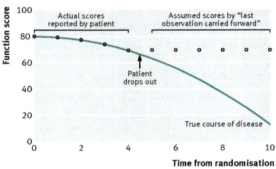

Fig Function scores over time for patient with chronic degenerative disease

Table Analysis of shoulder pain trial with three statistical methods

Analysis	Effect of acupuncture—difference in points (95% CI)	Standard error	P value
Available case	14.2 (5.1 to 23.4)	4.53	0.003
Last observation carried forward*	12.6 (3.9 to 21.3)	4.33	0.005
Multiple imputation†	14.3 (5.4 to 23.3)	4.45	0.002

*Missing final value replaced by baseline value (n=7).
†Using baseline score and treatment group.

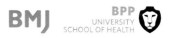

that may raise concerns about bias. Above all, analysis of missing data teaches us the importance of avoiding missing data in the first place: an informed guess, even using a technique as sophisticated as multiple imputation, is still a guess.

Contributors: AJV and DGA jointly wrote and agreed the text.

Competing interests: All authors have completed the ICMJE uniform disclosure form at www.icmje.org/coi_disclosure.pdf (available on request from the corresponding author) and declare: no support from any organisation for the submitted work; no financial relationships with any organisations that might have an interest in the submitted work in the previous three years; no other relationships or activities that could appear to have influenced the submitted work.

Provenance and peer review: Not commissioned; not externally peer reviewed.

1   Altman DG, Bland JM. Missing data. *BMJ* 2007;334:424.
2   Vickers AJ, Altman DG. Statistics notes: analysing controlled trials with baseline and follow up measurements. *BMJ* 2001;323:1123-4.
3   Molnar FJ, Man-Son-Hing M, Hutton B, Fergusson DA. Have last-observation-carried-forward analyses caused us to favour more toxic dementia therapies over less toxic alternatives? A systematic review. *Open Med* 2009;3:e31-50.
4   Bland JM, Altman DG. Regression towards the mean. *BMJ* 1994;308:1499.
5   Sterne JA, White IR, Carlin JB, Spratt M, Royston P, Kenward MG, et al. Multiple imputation for missing data in epidemiological and clinical research: potential and pitfalls. *BMJ* 2009;338:b2393.
6   White IR, Royston P, Wood AM. Multiple imputation using chained equations: issues and guidance for practice. *Stat Med* 2011;30:377-99.
7   White IR, Horton NJ, Carpenter J, Pocock SJ. Strategy for intention to treat analysis in randomised trials with missing outcome data. *BMJ* 2011;342:d40.

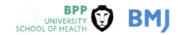

Strategy for intention to treat analysis in randomised trials with missing outcome dat

Ian R White, senior statistician[1], Nicholas J Horton, associate professor of mathematics and statistics[2], James Carpenter, reader in medical and social statistics[3], Stuart J Pococ[3] professor of medical statistics[3]

[1]MRC Biostatistics Unit, Cambridge CB2 0SR, UK

[2]Department of Mathematics and Statistics, Smith College, Clark Science Center, Northampton, MA 01063-0001, USA

[3]Department of Medical Statistics, London School of Hygiene and Tropical Medicine, London WC1E 7HT, UK

Correspondence to: I RWhite ian. white@mrc-bsu.cam.ac.uk

Cite this as: BMJ 2011;342:d40

DOI: 10.1136/bmj.d40

http://www.bmj.com/content/342/ bmj.d40

The intention to treat principle requires all participants in a clinical trial to be included in the analysis in the groups to which they were randomised, regardless of any departures from randomised treatment.[1] This principle is a key defence against bias, since participants who depart from randomised treatment are usually a non-random subset whose exclusion can lead to serious selection bias.[2]

However, it is unclear how to apply the intention to treat principle when investigators are unable to follow up all randomised participants. Filling in (imputing) the missing values is often seen as the only alternative to omitting participants from the analysis.[3] In particular, imputing by "last observation carried forward" is widely used,[4] but this approach has serious drawbacks.[3] For example, last observation carried forward was applied in a recent trial of a novel drug treatment in Alzheimer's disease.[5] The analysis was criticised because it effectively assumed that loss to follow-up halts disease progression,[6] but the authors argued that their analysis was in fact conservative.[7] Increasingly, trialists are expected to justify their handling of missing data and not simply rely on techniques that have been used in other clinical contexts.[8]

To guide investigators dealing with these tricky issues, we propose a four point framework for dealing with incomplete observations (box). Our aim is not to describe specific methods for analysing missing data, since these are described elsewhere,[9] [10] but to provide the framework within which methods can be chosen and implemented. We argue that all observed data should be included in the analysis, but undue focus on including all randomised participants can be unhelpful because participants with no post-randomisation data can contribute to the results only through untestable assumptions. The key issue is therefore not how to include all participants but what assumptions about the missing data are most plausibly correct, and how to perform appropriate analyses based on these assumptions. We now expand on these four points.

Attempt to follow up all randomised participants

Following up participants who withdraw from randomised treatment can be difficult but is important because they may differ systematically from those who remain on treatment. A trial that does not attempt to follow participants after treatment withdrawal cannot claim to follow the intention to treat principle.

Perform a plausible main analysis

When data are incomplete, all statistical analyses make untestable assumptions. The main analysis should be chosen to be valid under a plausible assumption about the missing data. For example, in the trial in Alzheimer's disease, consider a group of participants who are lost to follow-up between 6 and 12 months and a group of participants whose outcomes up to 6 months are similar to the first

ABSTRACT

Loss to follow-up is often hard to avoid in randomised trials. This article suggests a framework for intention to treat analysis that depends on making plausible assumptions about the missing data and including all participants in sensitivity analyses

group's but who are followed at least to 12 months. It r be reasonable to assume in the main analysis that th two groups have similar changes on average from 6 to months—a "missing at random" assumption, under wh an analysis of all observed outcome data, with adjustm for selected covariates, is appropriate. A similar assump underlies standard analyses of time to event data.

Possible analysis methods under a "missing at rand assumption include multiple imputation, inverse probabi weighting, and mixed models. These methods, and ot methods whose assumptions are less clear, are review elsewhere.[9] [10]

Assumptions about the missing data can often be suppo by collecting and reporting suitable information. For exam "missing at random" is often plausible if the reason for m missing data is shown to be administrative error but implaus if the reason is undocumented disease progression.

Perform sensitivity analyses

Good sensitivity analyses directly explore the eff of departures from the assumption made in the m analysis.[11] For example, if the main analysis assur similarity between groups who are and are not lost follow-up, a good sensitivity analysis might assume t the group who are lost to follow-up have systematic worse outcomes. A clinically plausible amount could added to or subtracted from imputed outcomes, possi using a technique such as multiple imputation.[9] Convers analysts could report how large an amount should added to or subtracted from imputed outcomes with changing the clinical interpretation of the trial. With a sn proportion of missing binary outcomes, best and worst c analyses may be appropriate.[12]

Results of the sensitivity analyses should be concis reported in a paper's abstract, saying, for example, whet the significance of the main analysis was maintained in sensitivity analyses or was changed in a limited or la number of sensitivity analyses.

Account for all randomised participants in the sensitivi analyses

When sensitivity analyses are carried out in this w they should account for all randomised participants. example, if a sensitivity analysis assumes a systema difference between missing and observed values, then results directly depend on the extent of missing data in t two trial arms.

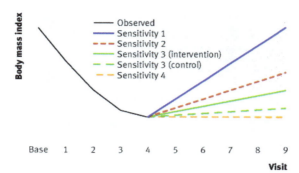

Fig Possible ways to impute outcome measures at visit 9 for a hypothetical participant in the obesity trial who drops out after visit 4: main analysis (last value brought forward) and three sensitivity analyses (1 assumes participants lost to follow-up return to baseline weight; 2 assumes 50% of weight regained, and 3 assumes intervention group regains a greater proportion of weight than controls)

Example of strategy in action

We illustrate the proposed strategy for intention to treat analysis using a recent trial comparing four doses of a new drug for obesity with two control groups.[13] Participants had nine planned visits over 20 weeks. The trial report suggests that participants who withdrew from trial treatment were followed up (point 1 of our proposed strategy). The primary analysis (point 2) used last observation carried forward in a "modified intention to treat" population that excluded three participants with no post-randomisation measures. A sensitivity analysis used repeated measures and thus assumed the data were missing at random. Since the main analysis implicitly assumes that participants neither gained nor lost weight on average after loss to follow-up, more direct approaches to sensitivity analysis are preferable. The figure shows our proposals for a hypothetical participant who attends only four of the nine visits (solid line). The red broken line shows the imputed value under last observation carried forward, the study authors' main analysis, while the other lines show three sensitivity analyses (point 3): sensitivity 1 shows the imputed value assuming that participants lost to follow-up returned to their baseline weight[14]; sensitivity 2 assumes they regained 50% of their lost weight; and sensitivity 3 assumes a larger fraction of the lost weight was regained in the intervention group.[15] Participants with no post-randomisation measures could be included in these analyses by making similar assumptions about their weight gain (point 4).

Discussion

The ideal solution to the problems discussed here is to avoid missing data altogether. This is rarely practical, but missing data can be minimised by careful design and trial management,[10] and in particular by attempting to follow up all participants.

The obesity trial illustrated our strategy applied to a trial with a repeatedly measured outcome. Analysis choices are more limited in trials with a singly measured outcome. In trials with time to event outcomes, an analysis that includes all randomised participants with censoring at the point of loss to follow-up is generally acceptable, but possible biases from informative censoring should be considered. In general, primary and sensitivity analyses should be specified in detail, ideally in the registered trial protocol and certainly before the unblinded data are seen, as a defence against claims of data driven changes to the analysis.[16]

Some argue for conser⸺ methods that are conservati⸺ conservative in others. For f⸺ forward is often claimed t⸺ biased in favour of a new treat⸺ suggested that authors should make the⸺ assumptions the basis for their primary analysis ⸺ provide conservatism by assessing sensitivity to departure⸺ from those assumptions.

Our proposed analysis strategy conforms to the intention to treat principle in the presence of missing outcomes and clarifies uncertainty regarding its application. It acknowledges the uncertainty introduced by missing data and therefore gives investigators an added incentive to minimise the extent of missing data.[19] Such guidelines are needed given the importance placed on intention to treat analyses and the ubiquity of missing data in real world clinical trials.

STRATEGY FOR INTENTION TO TREAT ANALYSIS WITH INCOMPLETE OBSERVATIONS

- 1. Attempt to follow up all randomised participants, even if they withdraw from allocated treatment
- 2. Perform a main analysis of all observed data that are valid under a plausible assumption about the missing data
- 3. Perform sensitivity analyses to explore the effect of departures from the assumption made in the main analysis
- 4. Account for all randomised participants, at least in the sensitivity analyses

---

Contributors: IRW had the original idea and wrote the first draft. All authors developed the idea, revised the paper and approved the final version. IRW is guarantor.

Funding: IRW was funded by MRC grant U.1052.00.006, NJH by NIH grant 5R01MH054693-11, and JC by ESRC Research Fellowship RES-063-27-0257.

Competing interests All authors have completed the unified competing interest form at www.icmje.org/coi_disclosure.pdf (available on request from the corresponding author) and declare no support from any organisation for the submitted work; JC has undertaken paid consultancy for various drug companies; and no other relationships or activities that could appear to have influenced the submitted work.

1   Moher D, Hopewell S, Schulz KF, Montori V, Gotzsche PC, Devereaux PJ, et al. CONSORT 2010 explanation and elaboration: updated guidelines for reporting parallel group randomised trials. *BMJ* 2010;340:c689.
2   Peduzzi P, Wittes J, Detre K. Analysis as randomised and the problem of non-adherence: an example from the Veterans Affairs randomized trial of coronary artery bypass surgery. *Stat Med* 1993;12:1185-95.
3   Altman D. Missing outcomes in randomized trials: addressing the dilemma. *Open Med* 2009;3(2):e51.
4   Committee for Proprietary Medicinal Products. *Points to consider on missing data*. 2001. www.emea.europa.eu/pdfs/human/ewp/177699EN.pdf.
5   Doody R, Gavrilova S, Sano M, Thomas R, Aisen P, Bachurin S, et al. Effect of dimebon on cognition, activities of daily living, behaviour, and global function in patients with mild-to-moderate Alzheimer's disease: a randomised, double-blind, placebo-controlled study. *Lancet* 2008;372:207-15.
6   Mackinnon A. Statistical treatment of withdrawal in trials of anti-dementia drugs. *Lancet* 2008;372:1382-3.
7   Doody R, Seely L, Thomas R, Sano M, Aisen P. Authors' reply. *Lancet* 2008;372:1383.
8   Sterne JAC, White IR, Carlin JB, Spratt M, Royston P, Kenward MG, et al. Multiple imputation for missing data in epidemiological and clinical research: potential and pitfalls. *BMJ* 2009;338:b2393.
9   Carpenter JR, Kenward MG. *Missing data in clinical trials — a practical guide*. Birmingham: National Institute for Health Research, 2008. www.pcpoh.bham.ac.uk/publichealth/methodology/projects/RM03_JH17_MK.shtml.
10   National Research Council. The prevention and treatment of missing data in clinical trials. 2010. www.nap.edu/catalog.php?record_id=12955.
11   Kenward MG, Goetghebeur EJT, Molenberghs G. Sensitivity analysis for incomplete categorical tables. *Stat Model* 2001;50:15-29.

12 Hollis S. A graphical sensitivity analysis for clinical trials with non-ignorable missing binary outcome. *Stat Med* 2002;21:3823-34.

13 Astrup A, Rössner S, Van Gaal L, Rissanen A, Niskanen L, Al Hakim M, et al. Effects of liraglutide in the treatment of obesity: a randomised, double-blind, placebo-controlled study. *Lancet* 2009;374:1606-16.

14 Ware JH. Interpreting incomplete data in studies of diet and weight loss. *N Engl J Med* 2003;348:2136-7.

15 White IR, Carpenter J, Evans S, Schroter S. Eliciting and using expert opinions about non-response bias in randomised controlled trials. *Clin Trials* 2007;4:125-39.

16 Shih WJ. Problems in dealing with missing data and informative censoring in clinical trials. *Curr Contr Trials Cardiovasc Med* 2002;3:4.

17 European Medicines Agency. Guideline on missing data in confirmatory clinical trials. 2010. www.ema.europa.eu/docs/en_GB/document_library/Scientific_guideline/2010/09/WC500096793.pdf.

18 Siddiqui O, Hung HM, O'Neill R. MMRM vs. LOCF: a comprehensive comparison based on simulation study and 25 NDA datasets. *J Biopharm Stat* 2009;19:227-46.

19 Wittes J. Missing inaction: preventing missing outcome data in randomized clinical trials. *J Biopharm Stat* 2009;19:957-68.

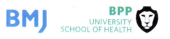

Multiple imputation for missing data in epidemiological and clinical research: potential and pitfalls

Jonathan A C Sterne, professor of medical statistics and epidemiology[1], Ian R White, senior scientist[2], John B Carlin, director of clinical epidemiology and biostatistics unit[3], Michael Spratt, research associate[1], Patrick Royston, senior scientist[4], Michael G Kenward, professor of biostatistics[5], Angela M Wood, lecturer in biostatistics[6], James R Carpenter, reader in medical and social statistics[5]

artment of Social Medicine,
ersity of Bristol, Bristol BS8

C Biostatistics Unit, Institute of
ic Health, Cambridge CB2 oSR

cal Epidemiology and
tatistics Unit, Murdoch
lren's Research Institute, and
ersity of Melbourne, Parkville,
ria 3052, Australia

cer and Statistical
hodology Groups, MRC Clinical
s Unit, London NW1 2DA

dical Statistics Unit, London
ol of Hygiene and Tropical
icine London, WC1E 7HT

artment of Public Health and
ary Care, Institute of Public
th, Cambridge

spondence to: J A C Sterne
han.sterne@bristol.ac.uk

this as: *BMJ* 2009;338:b2393

10.1136/bmj.b2393

//www.bmj.com/content/338/
02393

Missing data are unavoidable in epidemiological and clinical research but their potential to undermine the validity of research results has often been overlooked in the medical literature.[1] This is partly because statistical methods that can tackle problems arising from missing data have, until recently, not been readily accessible to medical researchers. However, multiple imputation—a relatively flexible, general purpose approach to dealing with missing data—is now available in standard statistical software,[2 3 4 5] making it possible to handle missing data semiroutinely. Results based on this computationally intensive method are increasingly reported, but it needs to be applied carefully to avoid misleading conclusions.

In this article, we review the reasons why missing data may lead to bias and loss of information in epidemiological and clinical research. We discuss the circumstances in which multiple imputation may help by reducing bias or increasing precision, as well as describing potential pitfalls in its application. Finally, we describe the recent use and reporting of analyses using multiple imputation in general medical journals, and suggest guidelines for the conduct and reporting of such analyses.

Consequences of missing data

Researchers usually address missing data by including in the analysis only complete cases —those individuals who have no missing data in any of the variables required for that analysis. However, results of such analyses can be biased. Furthermore, the cumulative effect of missing data in several variables often leads to exclusion of a substantial proportion of the original sample, which in turn causes a substantial loss of precision and power.

The risk of bias due to missing data depends on the reasons why data are missing. Reasons for missing data are commonly classified as: missing completely at random (MCAR), missing at random (MAR), and missing not at random (MNAR) (box 1).[6] This nomenclature is widely used, even though the phrases convey little about their technical meaning and practical implications, which can be subtle. When it is plausible that data are missing at random, but not completely at random, analyses based on complete cases may be biased. Such biases can be overcome using methods such as multiple imputation that allow individuals with incomplete data to be included in analyses. Unfortunately, it is not possible to distinguish between missing at random and missing not at random using observed data. Therefore, biases caused by data that are missing not at random can be addressed only by sensitivity analyses examining the effect of different assumptions about the missing data mechanism.

ABSTRACT

Most studies have some missing data. **Jonathan Sterne and colleagues** describe the appropriate use and reporting of the multiple imputation approach to dealing with them

Statistical methods to handle missing data

A variety of ad hoc approaches are commonly used to deal with missing data. These include replacing missing values with values imputed from the observed data (for example, the mean of the observed values), using a missing category indicator,[7] and replacing missing values with the last measured value (last value carried forward).[8] None of these approaches is statistically valid in general, and they can lead to serious bias. Single imputation of missing values usually causes standard errors to be too small, since it fails to account for the fact that we are uncertain about the missing values.

When there are missing outcome data in a randomised controlled trial, a common sensitivity analysis is to explore "best" and "worst" case scenarios by replacing missing values with "good" outcomes in one group and "bad" outcomes in the other group. This can be useful if there are only a few missing values of a binary outcome, but because imputing all missing values to good or bad is a strong assumption the sensitivity analyses can give a very wide range of estimates of the intervention effect, even if there are only a moderate number of missing outcomes. When outcomes are quantitative (numerical) such sensitivity analyses are not possible because there is no obvious good or bad outcome.

There are circumstances in which analyses of complete cases will not lead to bias. When missing data occur only in an outcome variable that is measured once in each individual, then such analyses will not be biased, provided that all variables associated with the outcome being missing can be included as covariates (under a missing at random assumption). Missing data in predictor variables also do not cause bias in analyses of complete cases if the reasons for the missing data are unrelated to the outcome.[9 10] In these circumstances, specialist methods to address missing data may lessen the loss of precision and power resulting from exclusion of individuals with incomplete predictor variables but are not required in order to avoid bias.

If we assume data are missing at random (box 1), then unbiased and statistically more powerful analyses (compared with analyses based on complete cases) can generally be done by including individuals with incomplete data. Sometimes this is possible by building a more general

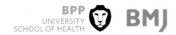

model incorporating information on partially observed variables—for example, using random effects models to incorporate information on partially observed variables from intermediate time points[11] [12] or by using bayesian methods to incorporate partially observed variables into a full statistical model from which the analysis of interest can be derived.[13] Other approaches include weighting the analysis to allow for the missing data,[14] [15] and maximum likelihood estimation that simultaneously models the reasons for missing data and the associations of interest in the substantive analysis.[13] Here, we focus on multiple imputation, which is a popular alternative to these approaches.

What is multiple imputation?

Multiple imputation is a general approach to the problem of missing data that is available in several commonly used statistical packages. It aims to allow for the uncertainty about the missing data by creating several different plausible imputed data sets and appropriately combining results obtained from each of them.

The first stage is to create multiple copies of the dataset, with the missing values replaced by imputed values. These are sampled from their predictive distribution based on the observed data—thus multiple imputation is based on a bayesian approach. The imputation procedure must fully account for all uncertainty in predicting the missing values by injecting appropriate variability into the multiple imputed values; we can never know the true values of the missing data.

The second stage is to use standard statistical methods to fit the model of interest to each of the imputed datasets. Estimated associations in each of the imputed datasets will differ because of the variation introduced in the imputation of the missing values, and they are only useful when averaged together to give overall estimated associations. Standard errors are calculated using Rubin's rules,[16] which take account of the variability in results between the imputed datasets, reflecting the uncertainty associated with the missing values. Valid inferences are obtained because we are averaging over the distribution of the missing data given the observed data.

Consider, for example, a study investigating the association of systolic blood pressure with the risk of subsequent coronary heart disease, in which data on systolic blood pressure are missing for some people. The probability that systolic blood pressure is missing is likely to decrease with age (doctors are more likely to measure it in older people), increasing body mass index, and history

of smoking (doctors are more likely to measure it in peo with heart disease risk factors or comorbidities). If assume that data are missing at random and that we h systolic blood pressure data on a representative sample individuals within strata of age, smoking, body mass ind and coronary heart disease, then we can use mult imputation to estimate the overall association betw systolic blood pressure and coronary heart disease.

Multiple imputation has potential to improve the vali of medical research. However, the multiple imputat procedure requires the user to model the distribution of e variable with missing values, in terms of the observed da The validity of results from multiple imputation depe on such modelling being done carefully and appropriat Multiple imputation should not be regarded as a rou technique to be applied at the push of a button—whene possible specialist statistical help should be obtained.

Pitfalls in multiple imputation analyses

A recent *BMJ* article reported the development of QRISK tool for cardiovascular risk prediction, based o large general practice research database.[17] The research correctly identified a difficulty with missing data in t database and used multiple imputation to handle missing data in their analysis. In their published predict model, however, cardiovascular risk was found to unrelated to cholesterol (coded as the ratio of total to h density lipoprotein cholesterol), which was surprisir The authors have subsequently clarified that when t restricted their analysis to individuals with comp information (no missing data) there was a clear associat between cholesterol and cardiovascular risk. Furthermor similar result was obtained after using a revised, improv imputation procedure.[19] It is thus important to be aware problems that can occur in multiple imputation analys which we discuss below.

Omitting the outcome variable from the imputation procedure

Often an analysis explores the association between one more predictors and an outcome but some of the predic have missing values. In this case, the outcome car information about the missing values of the predictors this information must be used.[20] For example, consi a survival model relating systolic blood pressure to t to coronary heart disease, fitted to data that have so missing values of systolic blood pressure. When miss systolic blood pressure values are imputed, individuals v develop coronary heart disease should have larger valu on average, than those who remain disease free. Failure include the coronary heart disease outcome and time to outcome when imputing the missing systolic blood press values would falsely weaken the association betwe systolic blood pressure and coronary heart disease.

Dealing with non-normally distributed variables

Many multiple imputation procedures assume that data normally distributed, so including non-normally distribu variables may introduce bias. For example, if a biochem factor had a highly skewed distribution but was implic assumed to be normally distributed, then imputat procedures could produce some implausibly low or e negative values. A pragmatic approach here is to transf such variables to approximate normality before imputat and then transform the imputed values back to the origi scale. Different problems arise when data are missing

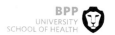

BOX 2 GUIDELINES FOR REPORTING ANY ANALYSIS POTENTIALLY AFFECTED BY MISSING DATA

Report the number of missing values for each variable of interest, or the number of cases with complete data for each important component of the analysis. Give reasons for missing values if possible, and indicate how many individuals were excluded because of missing data when reporting the flow of participants through the study. If possible, describe reasons for missing data in terms of other variables (rather than just reporting a universal reason such as treatment failure)

Clarify whether there are important differences between individuals with complete and incomplete data—for example, by providing a table comparing the distributions of key exposure and outcome variables in these different groups

Describe the type of analysis used to account for missing data (eg, multiple imputation), and the assumptions that were made (eg, missing at random)

For analyses based on multiple imputation

Provide details of the imputation modelling:

Report details of the software used and of key settings for the imputation modelling

Report the number of imputed datasets that were created (Although five imputed datasets have been suggested to be sufficient on theoretical grounds,[10] [11] a larger number (at least 20) may be preferable to reduce sampling variability from the imputation process[29])

What variables were included in the imputation procedure?

How were non-normally distributed and binary/categorical variables dealt with?

If statistical interactions were included in the final analyses, were they also included in imputation models?

If a large fraction of the data is imputed, compare observed and imputed values

Where possible, provide results from analyses restricted to complete cases, for comparison with results based on multiple imputation. If there are important differences between the results, suggest explanations, bearing in mind that analyses of complete cases may suffer more chance variation, and that under the missing at random assumption multiple imputation should correct biases that may arise in complete cases analyses

Discuss whether the variables included in the imputation model make the missing at random assumption plausible

It is also desirable to investigate the robustness of key inferences to possible departures from the missing at random assumption, by assuming a range of missing not at random mechanisms in sensitivity analyses. This is an area of ongoing research[30] [31]

---

binary or categorical variables. Some procedures[21] may handle these types of missing data better than others,[13] and this area requires further research.[22] [23]

Plausibility of missing at random assumption

"Missing at random" is an assumption that justifies the analysis, not a property of the data. For example, the missing at random assumption may be reasonable if a variable that is predictive of missing data in a covariate of interest is included in the imputation model, but not if the variable is omitted from the model. Multiple imputation analyses will avoid bias only if enough variables predictive of missing values are included in the imputation model. For example, if individuals with high socioeconomic status are both more likely to have their systolic blood pressure measured and less likely to have high systolic blood pressure then, unless socioeconomic status is included in the model used when imputing systolic blood pressure, multiple imputation will underestimate mean systolic blood pressure and may wrongly estimate the association between systolic blood pressure and coronary heart disease.

It is sensible to include a wide range of variables in imputation models, including all variables in the substantive analysis, plus, as far as computationally feasible, all variables predictive of the missing values themselves and all variables influencing the process causing the missing data, even if they are not of interest in the substantive analysis.[24] Failure to do so may mean that the missing at random assumption is not plausible and that the results of the substantive analysis are biased.

Data that are missing not at random

Some data are inherently missing not at random because it is not possible to account for systematic differences between the missing values and the observed values using the observed data. In such cases multiple imputation may give misleading results. For example, consider a study investigating predictors of depression. If individuals are more likely to miss appointments because they are depressed on the day of the appointment, then it may be impossible to make the missing at random assumption plausible, even if a large number of variables is included in the imputation model. When data are missing not at random, bias in analyses based on multiple imputation may be as big as or bigger than the bias in analyses of complete cases. Unfortunately, it is impossible to determine from the data how large a problem this may be. The onus rests on the data analyst to consider all the possible reasons for missing data and assess the likelihood of missing not at random being a serious concern.

Where complete cases and multiple imputation analyses give different results, the analyst should attempt to understand why, and this should be reported in publications.

Computational problems

Multiple imputation is computationally intensive and involves approximations. Some algorithms need to be run repeatedly in order to yield adequate results, and the required run length increases when more data are missing. Unforeseen difficulties may arise when the algorithms are run in settings different from those in which they were developed—for example, with high proportions of missing data, very large numbers of variables, or small numbers of observations. These points are discussed more fully elsewhere.[25]

Practical implications

The imputation models that were used in the original and revised versions of the QRISK cardiovascular risk prediction tool discussed above have been clarified.[26] The main reasons for the unexpected finding of a null association between cholesterol level and cardiovascular risk were omission of the cardiovascular disease outcome when imputing missing cholesterol values and calculation of the ratio of cholesterol to HDL based on imputed cholesterol and HDL values, which led to extreme values of the ratio being included in estimations. The impact of these pitfalls was increased by the high proportion of missing data (70% of HDL cholesterol values were missing).

Reporting in recent literature

Multiple imputation usually involves much more complicated statistical modelling than the single regression analyses commonly reported in medical research papers. However, constraints on the length of medical research papers mean that the details of the imputation procedures are often reported briefly, or not at all. Peer reviewers' lack of familiarity with multiple imputation may make it difficult for them to ask appropriate questions about the methods employed.

To examine recent use and reporting of multiple imputation, we searched four major general medical journals (*New England Journal of Medicine*, *Lancet*, *BMJ*, and *JAMA*) from 2002 to 2007 for articles reporting original research findings in which multiple imputation had been used. Articles were located by using search facilities on each journal's website to search for the phrase "multiple

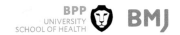

Table Reporting of multiple imputation in 59 papers published in general medical journals from 2002 to 2007*

Reported characteristic	No of papers
Amount of missing data	
No	23
Partially	6
Yes	30
Comparison of distribution of key variables in individuals with and without missing data	
No	52
Partially	2
Yes	5
No of imputations	
No	35
Yes	22
Unclear†	2
Results	
Both multiple imputation and complete case results tabulated	7
Multiple imputation results tabulated:	
Complete case results not reported	28
Complete case results in text	1
Complete case results stated to be similar	2
Complete case results tabulated:	
Multiple imputation results not reported‡	1
Multiple imputation results in text	4
Multiple imputation results stated to be similar	11
Stated no significant difference from multiple imputation	4
Sensitivity analysis done	1
Variables used in imputation	
No	53
No but normality discussed	1
Yes	5
Plausibility of the missing at random assumption	
No	56
Invalid discussion	2
Yes (sensitivity analysis)	1

*One paper that used multiple imputation to conduct sensitivity analyses rather than to deal with missing data was excluded from the table.

† Both papers used hotdeck imputation. One referred to a paper on multiple imputation but gave no further details, the other stated that "1000 imputation sequences" were used.

‡The methods section reports that a range of multiple imputation techniques were used to assess the robustness and sensitivity of conclusions, but no results are reported.

BOX 3 EXAMPLE OF USE OF MULTIPLE IMPUTATION

Burton et al[32] used data from a randomised controlled trial to compare the cost effectiveness of chemotherapy with that of standard palliative care in patients with advanced non-small cell lung cancer. Costs were obtained for a subset of 115 patients but were complete for only 82 patients. They gave the extent and distribution of missing data in table 1 of their paper. Patient and tumour characteristics were stated to be comparable in those with complete and incomplete data, but the effect of treatment on survival was stated to differ. The authors used the multiple imputation procedure in SAS statistical software (PROC MI) to impute the missing data. Variables included in the imputation models were listed. Five imputed datasets were created. A total run length of 12 500 iterations was used with imputations made after every 2500th imputation. Log and logit transformations were used to deal with non-normality, and a two stage procedure was used to deal with variables with a high proportion of zero values (semicontinuous distributions). Complete data were transformed back to their original scales before analysis.

The complete case analysis resulted in a higher mean cost for chemotherapy compared with palliative care (£2804 (€3285; $4580), 95% confidence interval £1236 to £4290) than did the analyses using multiple imputation (£2384, 95% CI £833 to £3954). The complete case analyses implied that chemotherapy was not cost effective (mean net monetary benefit −£3346), but the multiple imputation analyses implied that it was cost effective (mean net monetary benefit £1186), although confidence intervals were wide.

In the discussion, the authors noted the multiple imputation analysis "assumes that the incomplete cost data are missing at random such that the missingness of the cost components are associated only with the observed data, either the observed covariates or effectiveness." They did not, however, discuss whether the missing at random assumption was plausible or conduct sensitivity analyses investigating the robustness of the findings to assumed missing not at random mechanisms.

imputation" in the full text of all articles published duri the specified period. We found 59 articles, and the report use of multiple imputation roughly doubled over the years.

The table summarises the results of our survey. Vario methods for multiple imputation were used, with the speci method often reported only vaguely (for instance with book reference). Thirty six papers reported at least sor information on the amount of missing data, but only sev fully or partially reported comparisons of distributions key variables in individuals with and without missing da The number of imputation based datasets was reported 22 papers. Results of both imputed and complete cas analyses were fully reported in only seven papers, with o reporting sensitivity analyses. It was thus rarely possit to assess the impact of allowing for missing data. T variables used in imputation models were rarely listed, a the plausibility of the missing at random assumption w rarely assessed or discussed.

Suggested reporting guidelines

In the era of online supplements to research papers, it feasible and reasonable for authors to provide sufficie detail of imputation analyses to facilitate peer revie without distracting from the substantive research questio Box 2 lists the information that should be provided, eith as supplements or within the main paper. This exten guidance provided as part of the STROBE initiative strengthen the reporting of observational studies,[27] a complements suggestions for reporting of analyses usi multiple imputation in the epidemiological literature.[28]

Box 3 relates the suggested guidelines to the use multiple imputation in a published paper that examined t cost effectiveness of chemotherapy with that of standa palliative care in patients with advanced non-small cell lu cancer.

Summary

We are enthusiastic about the potential for multip imputation and other methods[14] to improve the valid of medical research results and to reduce the waste resources caused by missing data. The cost of multip imputation analyses is small compared with the co of collecting the data. It would be a pity if the avoidab pitfalls of multiple imputation slowed progress towards t wider use of these methods. It is no longer excusable missing values and the reason they arose to be swept und the carpet, nor for potentially misleading and inefficie analyses of complete cases to be considered adequate. hope that the pitfalls and guidelines discussed here w contribute to the appropriate use and reporting of metho to deal with missing data.

We thank Lucinda Billingham for checking our description of the article described in box 3.

Contributors: JACS, IRW, JBC, and JRC wrote the first draft of the paper. MS conducted the review of the use of multiple imputation medical journals and analysed the data. All authors contributed to the final draft and subsequent redrafts of the paper. JACS, IRW, and JRC will act as guarantors

Funding: Funded by UK Medical Research Council grant G0600599. IRW was supported by MRC grant U.1052.00.006 and JBC by NHMRC (Australia) grant 334336.

Competing interests: None declared.

Provenance and peer review: Not commissioned; externally peer reviewed.

1   Wood A, White IR, Thompson SG. Are missing outcome data adequately handled? A review of published randomised controlled trials. Clin Trials 2004;1:368-76.

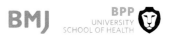

2   Royston P. Multiple imputation of missing values. *Stata J* 2004;4:227-41.

3   Royston P. Multiple imputation of missing values: update of ice. *Stata J* 2005;5:527-36.

4   Multiple Imputation Online. *Software* .www.multiple-imputation.com.

5   SAS Institute. *The MI procedure* . http://support.sas.com/rnd/app/papers/miv802.pdf.

6   Little RJ, Rubin DB. *Statistical analysis with missing data* . 2nd ed. New York: Wiley, 2002.

7   Vach W, Blettner M. Biased estimation of the odds ratio in case-control studies due to the use of ad hoc methods of correcting for missing values for confounding variables. *Am J Epidemiol* 1991;134:895-907.

8   Carpenter JR, Kenward MG. A critique of common approaches to missing data. In: *Missing data in randomised controlled trials— a practical guide* . Birmingham: National Institute for Health Research, 2008. www.pcpoh.bham.ac.uk/publichealth/methodology/projects/RM03_JH17_MK.shtml.

9   Steyerberg EW, van Veen M. Letter: Imputation is beneficial for handling missing data in predictive models. *J Clin Epidemiol* 2007;60:979.

10 Allison PD. Multiple imputation for missing data. A cautionary tale. *Sociol Methods Res* 2000;28:301-9.

11 Carpenter JR, Kenward MG. MAR methods for quantitative data. In: *Missing data in randomised controlled trials— a practical guide* . Birmingham: National Institute for Health Research, 2008. www.pcpoh.bham.ac.uk/publichealth/methodology/projects/RM03_JH17_MK.shtml.

12 Goldstein H, Carpenter J, Kenward MG, Levin K. Multilevel models with multivariate mixed response types. *Stat modelling* (in press).

13 Schafer JL. *Analysis of incomplete multivariate data* . London: Chapman and Hall, 1997.

14 Scharfstein DO, Rotnitzky A, Robins JM. Adjusting for non-ignorable drop-out using semiparametric non-response models. *J Am Stat Assoc* 1999;94:1096-120.

15 Carpenter JR, Kenward MG, Vansteelandt S. A comparison of multiple imputation and inverse probability weighting for analyses with missing data. *J R Stat Soc [Ser A]* 2006;169:571-84.

16 Rubin D. *Multiple imputation for nonresponse in surveys* . New York: Wiley, 1987.

17 Hippisley-Cox J, Coupland C, Vinogradova Y, Robson J, May M, Brindle P. Derivation and validation of QRISK, a new cardiovascular disease risk score for the United Kingdom: prospective open cohort study. *BMJ* 2007;335:136.

18 Peto R. Doubts about QRISK score: total/HDL cholesterol should be important [electronic response to Hippisley-Cox J, et al]. *BMJ* 2007 www.bmj.com/cgi/eletters/335/7611/136#172067.

19 Hippisley-Cox J, Coupland C, Vinogradova Y, Robson J, May M, Brindle P. QRISK— authors' response [electronic response]. *BMJ* 2007 www.bmj.com/cgi/eletters/335/7611/136#174181.

20 Moons KG, Donders RA, Stijnen T, Harrell FE. Using the outcome for imputation of missing predictor values was preferred. *J Clin Epidemiol* 2006;59:1092-101.

21 Van Buuren S, Boshuizen HC, Knook DL. Multiple imputation of missing blood pressure covariates in survival analysis. *Stat Med* 1999;18:681-94.

22 Horton NJ, Kleinman KP. Much ado about nothing: a comparison of missing data methods and software to fit incomplete data regression models. *Am Stat* 2007;61:79-90.

23 Bernaards CA, Belin TR, Schafer JL. Robustness of a multivariate normal approximation for imputation of incomplete binary data. *Stat Med* 2007;26:1368-82.

24 Collins LM, Schafer JL, Kam CM. A comparison of inclusive and restrictive strategies in modern missing data procedures. *Psychol Methods* 2001;6:330-51.

25 Carpenter J, Kenward M. *Brief comments on computational issues with multiple imputation* . www.missingdata.org.uk/mi_comp_issues.pdf.

26 Hippisley-Cox J, Coupland C, Vinogradova Y, Robson J, Brindle P. *QRISK cardiovascular disease risk prediction algorithm—comparison of the revised and the original analyses. Technical supplement 1* . 2007. www.qresearch.org/Public_Documents/QRISK1%20Technical%20Supplement.pdf.

27 Von Elm E, Altman DG, Egger M, Pocock SJ, Gøtzsche PC, Vandenbroucke JP, STROBE initiative. strengthening the reporting of observational studies in epidemiology (STROBE) statement: guidelines for reporting observational studies. *BMJ* 2007;335:806-8.

28 Klebanoff MA, Cole SR. Use of multiple imputation in the epidemiologic literature. *Am J Epidemiol* 2008;168:355-7.

29 Horton NJ, Lipsitz SR. Multiple imputation in practice: Comparison of software packages for regression models with missing variables. *Am Stat* 2001;55:244-54.

30 Demirtas H, Schafer JL. On the performance of random-coefficient pattern-mixture models for non-ignorable drop-out. *Stat Med* 2003;22:2553-75.

31 Carpenter JR, Kenward MG, White IR. Sensitivity analysis after multiple imputation under missing at random: a weighting approach. *Stat Methods Med Res* 2007;16:259-75.

32 Burton A, Billingham LJ, Bryan S. Cost-effectiveness in clinical trials: using multiple imputation to deal with incomplete cost data. *Clin Trials* 2007;4:154-61.

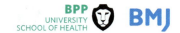

Assessing the value of diagnostic tests: a framework for designing and evaluating trials

Lavinia Ferrante di Ruffano, research fellow[1], Christopher J Hyde, professor of public health and clinical epidemiology[2], Kirsten J McCaffery, associate professor and principal research fellow[3], Patrick M M Bossuyt, professor of clinical epidemiology[4], Jonathan J Deeks, professor of biostatistics[1]

[1]Department of Public Health, Epidemiology, and Biostatistics, School of Health and Population Sciences, University of Birmingham, Birmingham B15 2TT, UK

[2]PenTAG, Institute for Health Services Research, Peninsula College of Medicine and Dentistry, University of Exeter, Exeter, UK

[3]Screening and Test Evaluation Program, School of Public Health, University of Sydney, Sydney, Australia

[4]Department of Clinical Epidemiology and Biostatistics, Academic Medical Centre, University of Amsterdam, Amsterdam, Netherlands

Correspondence to: Jonathan J Deeks
j.deeks@bham.ac.uk

Cite this as: BMJ 2012;344:e686

DOI: 10.1136/bmj.e686

http://www.bmj.com/content/344/bmj.e686

Most studies of diagnostic tests evaluate only their accuracy. Although such studies describe how well tests identify patients with disease (sensitivity) or without disease (specificity), further evidence is needed to determine a test's true clinical value. Firstly, since tests are rarely used in isolation, studies are needed that evaluate the performance of testing strategies, accounting for when and how a new test is used within a diagnostic pathway, and how its findings are combined with results of other tests.[1] Secondly, decision making involves selecting among multiple testing strategies; thus studies that compare test strategies and estimate differences in sensitivity and specificity are more informative than those that evaluate the accuracy of one test or diagnostic strategy.[2] Thirdly, improvements in test accuracy will not benefit patients unless they lead to changes in diagnoses and patient management, requiring evaluations of the effect of improved accuracy on decision making.[3] Finally, improved decision making is only one route by which tests affect patient health, and empirical evaluations are needed to compare the effect of test strategies on patient health.[4]

Ideally, new tests should only be introduced into clinical practice if evidence indicates that they have a better chance of improving patient health than existing tests.[5][6] Tests can be compared by evaluating the downstream consequences of testing on patient outcomes, either directly in a randomised controlled trial or by decision analysis models that integrate multiple sources of evidence. Test-treatment trials randomly allocate patients to tests, follow up subsequent management, and measure outcomes only after treatment has been received (fig 1).[7] Decision models use existing clinical data to extrapolate, through a number of assumptions, the link between intermediate outcomes (such as accuracy) and long term outcomes.[8] A key issue for trials and decision models is the selection of outcomes that need to be measured or modelled to evaluate how tests are

ABSTRACT

The value of a diagnostic test is not simply measured by its accuracy, but depends on how it affects patient health. This article presents a framework for the design and interpretation of studies that evaluate the health consequences of new diagnostic tests

affecting patients. This selection requires a priori knowle of the mechanisms by which tests affect patient health.

In this article, we provide a comprehensive review of mechanisms that can drive changes to patient health fr testing, and include a summary checklist to assist read researchers, and funders who wish to design or appra studies evaluating diagnostic tests. We have based framework on a review of a large cohort of published te treatment trials [9] and key methodological literature.

Effect of tests on patient health

To establish whether a new diagnostic test will cha health outcomes, it must be examined as part of a broa management strategy. Testing represents the first s of a test-treatment process: (1) a test is administered identify a target condition, (2) the test result is conside (3) alongside other evidence to decide a diagnosis, and a course of treatment is identified (5) and implemen (fig 2).[10]

Changes to any aspect of this pathway after introduction of a new test could trigger changes in hea outcomes. Table 1 lists the mechanisms that commo affect health outcomes.

Direct test effects

Test procedure

Some diagnostic procedures carry a risk of harm, hei alternatives that offer reduced procedural morbidity be of immediate benefit to patients. For example, use sentinel lymph node biopsy rather than dissection of axillary node to investigate metastatic spread in patie with early breast cancer results in much lower rates postoperative swelling of the arm, seroma formati numbness, and paraesthesia.[11]

Altering clinical decisions and actions

Feasibility and interpretability

The downstream value of a test will be impaired at outset if there are contraindications to its use or if it is pro to technical failure (feasibility), while tests that are m difficult to interpret (interpretability) could produce fev definitive results. Either problem could require additio

SUMMARY POINTS

- The value of diagnostic tests ultimately lies in their effect on patient outcomes
- Tests can affect patient health by changing diagnostic and treatment decisions, affecting time to treatment, modifying patient perceptions and behaviour, or putting patients at risk of direct harm
- Improved accuracy is not always a necessary prerequisite for improving patient health, nor does it guarantee other downstream improvements
- All elements of the management process (including decision making and treatment) must be considered when evaluating a diagnostic test
- Randomised controlled trials of tests can measure these processes directly to understand why and how changes to patient health have occurred

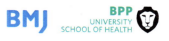

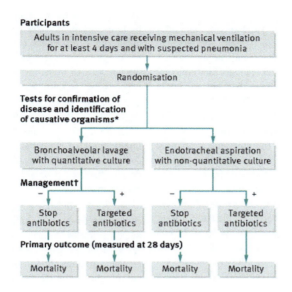

Fig 1 Design of a test-treatment randomised trial assessing whether bronchoalveolar lavage reduces the rate of death from ventilator associated pneumonia compared with endotracheal aspiration.[7] *All patients received broad spectrum antibiotics while waiting for test results. †In patients with confirmed pneumonia, antibiotics were adjusted using culture results and sensitivities; in test negative patients, antibiotics were discontinued

investigations, increasing the time to diagnosis, or reducing diagnostic and therapeutic yields through incorrect decision making or poor diagnostic confidence.

We observed this in a trial evaluating the diagnosis of coronary artery disease. Patients with acute chest pain who were allocated to exercise electrocardiography were significantly more likely to be referred for further

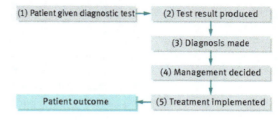

Fig 2 Simplified test-treatment pathway showing each component of a patient's management that can affect health outcomes[10]

investigation (coronary angiography) than those allocated to stress echocardiography.[12] This finding was caused by the higher frequency of inconclusive diagnoses produced by exercise electrocardiography, some of which were because the test was contraindicated.

Test accuracy, diagnostic yield, therapeutic yield, and treatment efficacy

More accurate tests will improve patient outcomes if the reductions in false positive or false negative results lead to more people receiving appropriate diagnoses (diagnostic yield) and appropriate treatment (therapeutic yield). The degree to which appropriate treatment can improve patient outcomes depends on its efficacy (treatment efficacy). In a trial evaluating the effect of fluorescence cystoscopy on the recurrence of bladder carcinoma in situ, the enhanced accuracy of fluorescence cystoscopy compared with white light cystoscopy alone led to a substantial increase in lesions being identified and treated at initial diagnosis, which significantly reduced the rate of recurrence.[13]

Diagnostic and therapeutic confidence

Although diagnostic yield generally increases with accuracy, it is also affected by a doctor's confidence in the diagnostic test. Tests inducing greater confidence could benefit patients by reducing the need for further investigations and shortening the time to treatment. The results of a trial evaluating the triage of patients with non-small cell lung cancer who were referred for operative staging with positron emission tomography (PET), show how a lack of diagnostic confidence can over-ride the benefits of improved accuracy.[14] PET identified patients for whom surgery was not indicated because of incurable mediastinal disease, but no difference was found in the proportion of patients avoiding a thoracotomy (the primary outcome) because surgeons still preferred to confirm PET findings using standard operative staging.

Doctors' confidence in the ensuing success of a treatment plan can affect treatment effectiveness by influencing the approach to treatment, particularly in surgery. Digital subtraction angiography (DSA) and multidetector row computed tomographic angiography (MDR-CTA) can both determine the location and degree of vascular narrowing in patients with symptomatic hardening of peripheral arteries. Doctors using DSA were significantly more confident of plans for surgery, owing to the test's clearer vascular images; however, MDR-CTA images were found to obscure interpretation and decrease confidence in the presence of vessel wall calcifications.[15]

Changing timeframes of decisions and actions

Tests that are undertaken earlier or produce results more quickly can improve health outcomes. For example, patients with unstable angina and non-ST segment elevated myocardial infarction allocated to receive early coronary

Table 1 Attributes of the test-treatment pathway that affect patient health

Pathway component and mechanism	Definition
Diagnostic test delivered	
Timing of test	Speed with which a test is performed within the management strategy
Feasibility	Completion of test process. Reasons for non-completion are: patient acceptability (patient's refusal to have test), test was contraindicated (clinical reason not to administer test), and technical failure (ability of diagnostic equipment to produce data)
Test process	Patients' interaction with test procedure, potentially causing physical or psychological harms or benefits
Test result produced	
Interpretability	Degree to which test data can be used to inform a diagnostic classification
Accuracy	Ability of a test to distinguish between patients who have disease and those who do not
Timing of results	Speed with which test results are available
Diagnosis made	
Timing of diagnosis	Speed with which a diagnostic decision is made
Diagnostic yield	Degree to which the test contributes to a patient diagnosis in any form, including: provision of a definitive diagnosis, confirmation of a suspected diagnosis, ruling out a working diagnosis, and distinguishing between alternative diagnoses with different treatment implications. Diagnostic yield is different from accuracy because it also incorporates any other information used by a doctor to make a diagnosis (such as previous test results)
Diagnostic confidence	Degree of confidence that doctors and patients have in the validity or applicability of a test result
Management decided	
Therapeutic yield	Degree to which diagnostic decisions affect treatment plans
Therapeutic confidence	Certainty with which doctors and patients pursue a course of treatment
Treatment implemented	
Timing of treatment	Speed with which patients receive treatment
Treatment efficacy	Ability of the treatment intervention to improve patient outcomes
Adherence	Extent to which patients participate in the management plan, as advised by their doctor, to attain therapeutic goal

angiography had a reduced risk of death, non-fatal cardiac events, and readmission.[16] Patients with ventilator associated pneumonia allocated to a rapid antimicrobial susceptibility test received definitive results on average 2.8 days earlier than those receiving the standard susceptibility test and experienced significantly fewer days of fever, bouts of diarrhoea, and days on mechanical ventilation.[17]

However, quicker results are beneficial only if they produce earlier diagnosis or treatment. The addition of polymerase chain reaction (PCR) to conventional analysis of nasopharyngeal swabs for distinguishing between viral and bacterial causes of lower respiratory tract infection failed to decrease time to treatment, because physicians were unwilling to base treatment decisions solely on PCR, preferring to wait for slower bacterial results.[18] Earlier diagnosis can provide psychological benefit by dispelling anxiety or providing earlier reassurance but can also cause psychological harm, particularly if effective treatments are unavailable. The psychosocial impacts of an earlier diagnosis have been highlighted in women following a positive cervical smear test[19] or mammogram.[20]

Influencing patient and clinician perceptions

The patient's perspective and the doctor's personal perspective can also influence decision making, sometimes in unexpected ways. These unpredictable responses can eliminate or enhance potential improvements gained from other aspects of the test-treatment pathway.

Patients

Patients' perceptions of testing, their experience of the testing process, and their understanding of the test result can all affect downstream health. Many studies show social, emotional, cognitive, and behavioural effects of testing across various clinical conditions.[21]

Test-treatment pathways will be unsuccessful if patients are unwilling to undergo a procedure. This is especially important if multiple testing is required; an unpleasant first test can adversely influence patients' willingness to attend follow-up testing or treatment. The experience of undergoing tests can also influence illness beliefs. In a randomised

trial, women who were able to observe their diagnos hysteroscopy on a screen were reportedly less optimis about the effectiveness of treatment offered, experienc more anxiety, but were better able to deal with procedu discomfort than women who could not see the screen.[22]

Diagnostic placebo effects might occur if the impressi of a thorough investigation improves perceptions of hea status. This could account for the significant improvemen in health utility that were reported by patients with acu undifferentiated chest pain diagnosed in a specialist un compared with those diagnosed in emergency departmen despite having equivalent treatment and rates of adver cardiac events.[23]

Receiving a diagnosis can have behavioural and hea consequences—for example, by confirming patien negative health beliefs. Patients with lower back pa reported higher pain scores and poorer health status aft receiving an x ray than those who received only a standa consultation.[24] The incidental diagnosis of non-patholog abnormalities may have given patients a reason for th pain and encouraged illness behaviour despite the absen of an organic cause.

Adherence to treatment

Patients' experiences and perceptions of the test-treatme pathway will also affect downstream health behaviou such as the willingness or motivation to adhere to medic advice.[25] Negative perceptions or experiences of testing a clinical diagnosis could cause patients to lose confidence the diagnosis or management plan, making them relucta to have subsequent testing or treatment.

Doctors

Doctors' emotional, cognitive, social, or behaviour perspectives, although external to objective medic concerns, are nevertheless important in decision makir Referring doctors might modify management to reassu and satisfy patients or to prevent perceived threats malpractice, often by requesting additional diagnos information.[26] This defensive medicine tends to rai the diagnostic threshold needed to trigger a change management,[27] and if additional tests are less accura harmful, or lead to treatment delays, patients will adversely affected.

Systemic approach to evaluating tests

These examples establish that diagnostic tests often affe patient health outcomes in many complex ways. Although te accuracy is commonly regarded as the main mechanism influence clinical effectiveness,[28] we caution against its u as a surrogate for patient health. Only by looking at the te treatment pathway as a whole can we identify which outcom need to be evaluated to fully capture a test's health effects.

Sound evaluations of healthcare demand explanati of how the intervention will improve patient health This is equally true of diagnostic tests, although they a considerably more challenging to evaluate because many intermediate, interacting factors are at stake. Th need to identify which of these factors will exert an effe and how, is a key tenet of complex intervention guidance Table 2 provides a list of questions to guide the structure assessment of which processes are relevant and need be measured within a given diagnostic comparison. Th approach highlights precisely where in a test-treatmen pathway important differences might originate, and will b useful for designing studies, appraising existing researc and determining what new evidence is needed to formula diagnostic guidelines (box).

Fig 3 Sample size calculations for test-treatment randomised controlled trials. In randomised trials of interventions, all participants in a study group are allocated to receive the same intervention. In test-treatment trials, participants in each group receive a variety of interventions, depending on the test results and ensuing diagnosis. The magnitude of the observed treatment effect depends on the differences in proportions of patients who receive interventions appropriate to their condition in each group. This proportion would be expected to be quite small. The figure identifies those participants who contribute statistical power in a randomised trial comparing two tests (where the difference in outcome originates entirely from a difference in diagnostic accuracy). Test 2 has higher sensitivity than test 1 (difference shown in A). Test 2 also has higher specificity than test 1 (difference shown in B). Different widths of diseased and non-diseased columns indicate the prevalence of disease in the study sample. Only participants in A and B would have different test results if they received test 2 rather than test 1 and therefore the potential for different outcomes (all other participants in the study would have the same test result, irrespective of which test they were allocated to). Statistical power therefore depends on only the numbers of participants in A and B (particularly A); for example, if disease prevalence was 20%, and test 2 improved sensitivity by 20%, only 4% of the total sample size would fall in A[34]

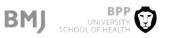

e 2 Checklist to determine clinically important differences between test-treatment pathways of new and existing diagnostic test strategies

st-treatment pathway		Questions	Yes/no	Notes	Outcome to capture difference
mponent	Mechanism				
Test delivery	**Timing of test**				
	Time to test delivery	Do the strategies provide testing within comparable timeframes (or does one strategy deliver a diagnostic test considerably earlier than the other)?			
	Feasibility				
	Acceptability	Is the new test likely to be as acceptable to patients as the existing test (or does one test cause increased discomfort, for example)?			
	Clinical con-traindications	Is the new test likely to be suitable in similar proportions of the relevant patient group (or will the new test be contraindicated in more or fewer patients than the existing test)?			
	Technical failure rates	Do the two tests produce similar proportions of failed procedures (or does the process of one test tend to fail more frequently than the other)?			
	Test process				
	Procedural harms or benefits	Are the two tests similar in how they affect patients during their application, physically or psychologically (or is one test more intrusive than the other or has a higher procedural morbidity than the other)?			
	Placebo effect	Does the new strategy give patients a similar perspective on being investigated (or could the new strategy encourage patients as to the thoroughness of their investigation)?			
Test result	Interpretability				
	Ease of interpretation	Do the two processes produce similar frequencies of clearly interpretable test results (or once completed successfully, does one test tend to produce a higher frequency of indeterminate or unreadable results than the other)?			
	Accuracy				
	Accuracy	Do the tests correctly identify the target condition in the same number of patients (or does one test correctly identify a higher proportion of patients with disease or without disease than the other)?			
	Timing of results				
	Time to produce a result	Is the speed with which results are processed similar between tests (or does the new test have a shorter turnaround time between testing and production of results than the existing test)?			
Diagnostic cision	**Timing of diagnosis**				
	Speed of diagnosis	Do the strategies produce diagnoses in comparable timeframes (or do patients given one test receive a diagnosis more quickly than patients given the other test)?			
	Diagnostic yield				
	Diagnoses made	Do the tests contribute to patient diagnosis to similar degrees (or do the results of one test tend to be given more weight than the other)?			
	Diagnostic confidence				
	Doctors' confidence in diagnosis	Is the degree of confidence that doctors have in the validity or applicability of a test result similar to that of its comparator test (or does a new test provide greater reassurance to doctors, or are its results considered less reliable by doctors)?			
	Patients' confidence in diagnosis	Is the degree of confidence that a patient has in the diagnostic process, or the diagnosis itself, likely to vary between strategies (or does a new test provide greater or lesser reassurance to patients, owing to doctors' confidence, the testing experience, or understanding of test results)?			
Treatment cision	**Therapeutic yield**				
	Treatment choices	Do the comparative tests contribute to the formulation of a management plan to similar degrees (or does one test lead to more patients receiving appropriate treatment than the other)?			

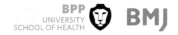

Test-treatment pathway		Questions	Yes/no	Notes	Outcome to capture difference
Component	Mechanism				
	Therapeutic confidence				
	Doctors' confidence in treatment choice	Do doctors have similar confidence in pursuing a treatment plan between intervention arms (or does a test improve treatment success)?			
	Patients' confidence in treatment choice	Do patients have similar confidence in treatment plans based on diagnostic testing (or does the new test improve patients' understanding of the choice in management)?			
(5) Treatment implementation	**Timing of treatment**				
	Time to treatment	Do the diagnostic strategies lead to patients receiving treatment within comparable timeframes (or do patients given one test receive treatment earlier than those given the other test)?			
	Treatment efficacy				
	Efficacy of treatment	Does use of the intervention in patients identified to have disease lead to improvements in patient outcomes (or is the intervention ineffective)?			
	Adherence				
	Adherence to treatment	Are patients as likely to adhere to treatment plans regardless of the test strategy used (or does one strategy lead to more refusals or poorer compliance with treatment)?			

BOX EXAMPLE EVALUATION OF A DIAGNOSTIC TEST

Consider replacing conventional imaging (which usually involves multiple images with different technologies) with PET-computed tomography (CT) for the diagnosis of breast cancer recurrence in adults with clinically suspected tumours. The first step is to state the alternative diagnostic and management pathways that will be compared, and to note the differences between them to narrow down mechanisms to consider.

How PET-CT improves patient health

On the basis of a recent systematic review, we might expect the improved accuracy of PET-CT to be the main mechanism driving changes to health.[31] A more accurate differentiation of patients with and without recurrence would increase diagnostic and therapeutic yields, and the treatment consequences thereof.

Accuracy improvements could be offset by other decisions; patient contraindications to PET-CT could mean patients must revert to the existing multitest strategy. Although the known technical capabilities of PET-CT might increase doctors' confidence, the obligation to rely on the results of one test could initially weaken such confidence, thus reducing the effective accuracy of the new protocol.

By contrast, use of a single test could accelerate treatment by enabling a quicker diagnosis. Nevertheless, the requirement for a specialist to interpret PET-CT scans could mitigate this benefit. Comparative procedural harms might also differ, highlighting the importance of considering direct health outcomes, although conventional imaging usually requires CT, so the exposure to radiation as a consequence of using PET-CT is probably similar. However, the success with which the new strategy operates will depend on any differences in perceptions and experiences; PET-CT might be more or less reassuring to patients and clinicians, and these unknown influences would need to be measured carefully.

Choosing outcomes to evaluate PET-CT

Using the framework prompts the consideration of informative outcomes by showing the new pathway's full range of health effects, and allowing the assessment of all relevant direct and downstream measures of important patient outcomes. In the present example, such outcomes might include measures of anxiety, reassurance, health beliefs, function, symptoms, recurrence, progression, and survival.

Identified mechanisms can be measured as process outcomes in order to assess whether the new pathway is operating as expected. For example, the impact of temporality could be assessed as the time to diagnosis or time to treatment, and diagnostic confidence might be measured directly or by the number of additional investigations ordered.

We identify three benefits from using this framework. Firstly, it presents a structure for carefully developing rationale that underpins the performance of a putative test strategy. Secondly, it guides the identification of outcomes for randomised controlled trials, and will also assist constructing appropriate decision models, particularly when trials are not practicable.[32] Finally, the approach supports full interpretation of empirical results by enabling trialists to distinguish between true ineffectiveness, poor protocol implementation, and methodological flaws in the study design.[33] These tasks are particularly important for trials of tests, where sample sizes often need to be several orders of magnitude larger than they do in trials of treatment to detect differences in patient outcomes (fig 3).[34] Findings of no effect are all too often interpreted as "evidence of absence," when in reality studies rarely make provision for being able to attribute negative results to the diagnostic intervention, the study design, or (importantly) inconsistently implemented test-treatment strategy. These interpretations can be distinguished by identifying and measuring the relevant driving mechanisms. By recording the use of additional diagnostic tests, treatments, and decision making, the failure of PET to reduce the rate of thoracotomies in patients with non-small cell lung cancer was shown to lie with an ill conceived treatment strategy rather than with efficacy of the test.[14] The trialists identified patients for whom PET, unexpectedly failed to change management decisions, and they then found that strong preferences for the existing management (to operate on all patients with stage IIIa disease) exceeded the effect of PET results. By identifying all relevant mechanisms, and measuring how they exert their effect, test-treatment trials are more likely to contribute important evidence to the use of tests in clinical practice.

Conclusion

Establishing benefit to patient health must be the priority for diagnostic evaluations. Test accuracy is one component of test evaluation, but does not capture the impact of test

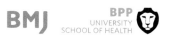

on patients. By considering the ways in which tests affect patients' health, we reiterate the complex intervention perspective[30] that it is not sufficient to measure outcomes, but rather it is essential to understand how these outputs are created, by conducting analyses of their workings and the mechanisms that underpin them. Clearly, this process must be undertaken with expert and stakeholder consultation to ensure all influential mechanisms are identified.

Contributors: JJD conceived the idea for this project with support from CJH. LFR did most of the primary research for the paper. The initial framework was devised by LFR, CJH, and JJD, and further refined by all authors. All the authors drafted, revised, and gave final approval to the article. JJD is the guarantor.

Funding: The development of the framework was funded partly by the UK Medical Research Council Methodology Programme (grant G0600545, awarded to JJD), as part of a wider investigation into the use of randomised trials for evaluating the clinical effectiveness of diagnostic tests. The funders had no involvement in the research project. JJD is partly supported by the Medical Research Council Midland Hub for Trials Methodology Research, University of Birmingham (grant G0800808).

Competing interests: All authors have completed the ICJME unified disclosure form at www.icmje.org/coi_disclosure.pdf and declare: the work was funded partly by the UK Medical Research Council Methodology Programme; no financial relationships with any organisations that might have an interest in the submitted work in the previous three years; and no other relationships or activities that could appear to have influenced the submitted work.

Provenance and peer review: Not commissioned; externally peer reviewed.

1 Bossuyt PM, Irwig L, Craig J, Glasziou P. Comparative accuracy: assessing new tests against existing diagnostic pathways. *BMJ* 2006;332:1089-92.

2 Leeflang MMG, Deeks JJ, Gatsonis C, Bossuyt PMM, on behalf of the Cochrane Diagnostic Test Accuracy Working Group. Systematic reviews of diagnostic test accuracy. *Ann Intern Med* 2008;149:889-97.

3 Fryback DG, Thornbury JR. The efficacy of diagnostic imaging. *Med Decis Making* 1991;11:88-94.

4 Lijmer JG, Bossuyt PMM. Various randomized designs can be used to evaluate medical tests. *J Clin Epidemiol* 2009;62:364-73.

5 Fineberg HV. Evaluation of computed tomography: achievement and challenge. *Am J Roentgenol* 1978;131:1-4.

6 Schünemann HJ, Oxman AD, Brozek J, Glasziou P, Jaeschke R, Vist GE, et al. Grading quality of evidence and strength of recommendations for diagnostic tests and strategies. *BMJ* 2008;336:1106-10.

7 Canadian Critical Care Trials Group. Randomized trial of diagnostic techniques for ventilator-associated pneumonia. *N Engl J Med* 2006;355:2619-30.

8 Sutton AJ, Cooper NJ, Goodacre S, Stevenson M. Integration of meta-analysis and economic decision modeling for evaluating diagnostic tests. *Med Decis Making* 2008;28:650-67.

9 Ferrante di Ruffano L, Davenport C, Eisinga A, Hyde C, Deeks JJ. A capture-recapture analysis demonstrated that randomized controlled trials evaluating the impact of diagnostic tests on patient outcomes are rare. *J Clin Epidemiol* 2012;65:282-7.

10 Bossuyt PMM, Lijmer JG. Traditional health outcomes in the evaluation of diagnostic tests. *Acad Radiol* 1999;6:S77-80.

11 Purushotham AD, Upponi S, Klevesath MB, Bobrow L, Millar K, Myles J, et al. Morbidity after sentinel lymph node biopsy in primary breast cancer: results from a randomized controlled trial. *J Clin Oncol* 2005;23:4312-21.

12 Jeetley P, Burden L, Senior R. Stress echocardiography is superior to exercise ECG in the risk stratification of patients presenting with acute chest pain with negative Troponin. *Eur J Echocardiogr* 2006;7:155-64.

13 Babjuk M, Soukup V, Petrík R, Jirsa M, Dvorácek J. 5-aminolaevulinic acid-induced fluorescence cystoscopy during transurethral resection reduces the risk of recurrence in stage Ta/T1 bladder cancer. *BJU Int* 2005;96:798-802.

14 Viney RC, Boyer MJ, King MT, Kenny PM, Pollicino CA, Mclean JM, et al. Randomized controlled trial of the role of positron emission tomography in the management of stage I and II non-small-cell lung cancer. *J Clin Oncol* 2004;22:2357-62.

15 Kock MC, Adriaensen ME, Pattynama PM, van Sambeek MR, van Urk H, Stijnen T, et al. DSA versus multi-detector row CT angiography in peripheral arterial disease: randomized controlled trial. *Radiology* 2005;237:727-37.

16 Cannon CP, Weintraub WS, Demopoulos LA, Vicari R, Frey MJ, Lakkis N, et al. Comparison of early invasive and conservative strategies in patients with unstable coronary syndromes treated with the glycoprotein IIb/IIIa inhibitor tirofiban. *N Engl J Med* 2001;344:1879-87.

17 Bouza E, Torres MV, Radice C, Cercenado E, de Diego R; Sánchez-Carrillo C, et al. Direct E-test (AB Biodisk) of respiratory samples improves antimicrobial use in ventilator-associated pneumonia. *Clin Infect Dis* 2007;44:382-7.

18 Oosterheert JJ, van Loon AM, Schuurman R, Hoepelman AI, Hak E, Thijsen S, et al. Impact of rapid detection of viral and atypical bacterial pathogens by real-time polymerase chain reaction for patients with lower respiratory tract infection. *Clin Infect Dis* 2005;41:1438-44.

19 McCaffery KJ, Irwig L, Turner R, Chan SF, Macaskill P, Lewicka M, et al. Psychosocial outcomes of three triage methods for the management of borderline abnormal cervical smears: an open randomised trial. *BMJ* 2010;340:b4491.

20 Barton MB, Morley DS, Moore S, Allen JD, Kleinman KP, Emmons KM et al. Decreasing women's anxieties after abnormal mammograms: a controlled trial. *J Natl Cancer Inst* 2004;96:529-38.

21 Bossuyt PMM, McCaffery K. Multiple pathways and additional patient outcomes in evaluations of testing. *Med Decis Making* 2009;29:E30-8.

22 Ogden J, Heinrich M, Potter C, Kent A, Jones S. The impact of viewing a hysteroscopy on a screen on the patient's experience: a randomised trial. *BJOG* 2009;116:286-93.

23 Goodacre SW, Nicholl J, Dixon S, Cross E, Angelini K, Arnold J, et al. Randomised controlled trial and economic evaluation of a chest pain observation unit compared with routine care. *BMJ* 2004;328:254-60.

24 Djais N, Kalim H. The role of lumbar spine radiography in the outcomes of patients with simple acute low back pain. *APLAR J Rheumatol* 2005;8:45-50.

25 Haynes RB, Ackloo E, Sahota N, McDonald HP, Yao X. Interventions for enhancing medication adherence. *Cochrane Database Syst Rev* 2008;2:CD000011.

26 Summerton, N. Positive and negative factors in defensive medicine: a questionnaire study of general practitioners. *BMJ* 1995;310:27-9.

27 Hauser MJ, Commons ML, Bursztajn HJ, Gutheil TG. Fear of malpractice liability and its role in clinical decision making. In: Gutheil TG, Bursztajn HJ, Brodsky A, Alexander V, eds. Decision making in psychiatry and the law. 1st ed. Williams and Wilkins, 1991.

28 Hunink MGM, Krestin GP. Study design for concurrent development, assessment, and implementation of new diagnostic imaging technology. *Radiology* . 2002;222:604-14.

29 Moher D, Hopewell S, Schultz KF, Montori V, Gøtzsche PC, Devereaux PJ, et al. CONSORT 2010 explanation and elaboration: updated guidelines for reporting parallel group randomised trials. *BMJ* 2010;340:c869.

30 Craig P, Dieppe P, Macintyre S, Michie S, Nazareth I, Petticrew M. Developing and evaluating complex interventions: new guidance. Medical Research Council, 2008.

31 Pennant M, Takwoingi Y, Pennant L, Davenport C, Fry-Smith A, Eisinga A, et al. A systematic review of positron emission tomography (PET) and positron emission tomography/computed tomography (PET/CT) for the diagnosis of breast cancer recurrence. *Health Technol Assess* 2010;14:1-103.

32 Pletcher MJ, Pignone M. Evaluating the clinical utility of a biomarker: a review of methods for estimating health impact. *Circulation* 2011;123:1116-24.

33 Rychetnik L, Frommer M, Hawe P, Shiell A. Criteria for evaluating evidence on public health interventions. *J Epidemiol Community Health* 2002;56:119-27.

34 Deeks JJ. Assessing outcomes following tests. In: Price CP, Christenson EH, eds. Evidence-based laboratory medicine: principles, practice and outcomes. 2nd ed. AACC Press; 2007;95-111.

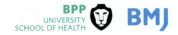

Three techniques for integrating data in mixed methods studies

Alicia O'Cathain, professor[1], Elizabeth Murphy, professor[2], Jon Nicholl, professor[1]

[1]Medical Care Research Unit, School of Health and Related Research, University of Sheffield, Sheffield S1 4DA, UK

[2]University of Leicester, Leicester, UK

Correspondence to: A O'Cathain
a.ocathain@sheffield.ac.uk

Cite this as: *BMJ* 2010;341:c4587

DOI: 10.1136/bmj.c4587

http://www.bmj.com/content/341/bmj.c4587

Health researchers are increasingly using designs that combine qualitative and quantitative methods, and this is often called mixed methods research.[1] Integration—the interaction or conversation between the qualitative and quantitative components of a study—is an important aspect of mixed methods research, and, indeed, is essential to some definitions.[2] Recent empirical studies of mixed methods research in health show, however, a lack of integration between components,[3 4] which limits the amount of knowledge that these types of studies generate. Without integration, the knowledge yield is equivalent to that from a qualitative study and a quantitative study undertaken independently, rather than achieving a "whole greater than the sum of the parts."[5]

Barriers to integration have been identified in both health and social research.[6 7] One barrier is the absence of formal education in mixed methods research. Fortunately, literature is rapidly expanding to fill this educational gap, including descriptions of how to integrate data and findings from qualitative and quantitative methods.[8 9] In this article we outline three techniques that may help health researchers to integrate data or findings in their mixed methods studies and show how these might enhance knowledge generated from this approach.

Triangulation protocol

Researchers will often use qualitative and quantitative methods to examine different aspects of an overall research question. For example, they might use a randomised controlled trial to assess the effectiveness of a healthcare intervention and semistructured interviews with patients and health professionals to consider the way in which the intervention was used in the real world. Alternatively, they might use a survey of service users to measure satisfaction with a service and focus groups to explore views of care in more depth. Data are collected and analysed separately for each component to produce two sets of findings. Researchers will then attempt to combine these findings, sometimes calling this process triangulation. The term triangulation can be confusing because it has two meanings.[10] It can be used to describe corroboration between two sets of findings or to describe a process of studying a problem using different methods to gain a more complete picture. The latter meaning is commonly used in mixed methods research and is the meaning used here.

ABSTRACT

Techniques designed to combine the results of qualitative and quantitative studies can provide researchers with more knowledge than separate analysis

The process of triangulating findings from differe methods takes place at the interpretation stage of study when both data sets have been analysed separate (figure). Several techniques have been described f triangulating findings. They require researchers to list t findings from each component of a study on the sar page and consider where findings from each method agr (convergence), offer complementary information on t same issue (complementarity), or appear to contradict ea other (discrepancy or dissonance).[11-13] Explicitly looking f disagreements between findings from different metho is an important part of this process. Disagreement is n a sign that something is wrong with a study. Explorati of any apparent "inter-method discrepancy" may lead a better understanding of the research question,[14] and range of approaches have been used within health servic research to explore inter-method discrepancy.[15]

The most detailed description of how to carry o triangulation is the triangulation protocol,[11] which althou developed for multiple qualitative methods, is relevant mixed methods studies. This technique involves produci a "convergence coding matrix" to display findings emergi from each component of a study on the same page. Th is followed by consideration of where there is agreemer partial agreement, silence, or dissonance between findin from different components. This technique for triangulati is the only one to include silence—where a theme or findi arises from one data set and not another. Silence might expected because of the strengths of different methods examine different aspects of a phenomenon, but surpri silences might also arise that help to increase understandi or lead to further investigations.

The triangulation protocol moves researchers fro thinking about the findings related to each method, to wh Farmer and colleagues call meta-themes that cut acro the findings from different methods.[11] They show a worke example of triangulation protocol, but we could find no oth published example. However, similar principles were use in an iterative mixed methods study to understand patie and carer satisfaction with a new primary angioplas service.[16] Researchers conducted semistructured interviev with 16 users and carers to explore their experiences ar views of the new service. These were used to develo a questionnaire for a survey of 595 patients (and 418 their carers) receiving either the new service or usual car Finally, 17 of the patients who expressed dissatisfactic with aftercare and rehabilitation were followed up explore this further in semistructured interviews. A shi of thinking to meta-themes led the researchers away fro reporting the findings from the interviews, survey, ar follow-up interviews sequentially to consider the met

SUMMARY POINTS

- Health researchers are increasingly using designs which combine qualitative and quantitative methods
- However, there is often lack of integration between methods
- Three techniques are described that can help researchers to integrate data from different components of a study: triangulation protocol, following a thread, and the mixed methods matrix
- Use of these methods will allow researchers to learn more from the information they have collected

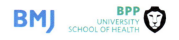

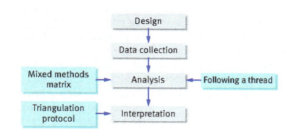

Fig Point of application for three techniques for integrating data in mixed methods research

themes of speed and efficiency, convenience of care, and discharge and after care. The survey identified that a higher percentage of carers of patients using the new service rated the convenience of visiting the hospital as poor than those using usual care. The interviews supported this concern about the new service, but also identified that the weight carers gave to this concern was low in the context of their family member's life being saved.

Morgan describes this move as the "third effort" because it occurs after analysis of the qualitative and the quantitative components.[17] It requires time and energy that must be planned into the study timetable. It is also useful to consider who will carry out the integration process. Farmer and colleagues require two researchers to work together during triangulation, which can be particularly important in mixed methods studies if different researchers take responsibility for the qualitative and quantitative components.[11]

Following a thread

Moran-Ellis and colleagues describe a different technique for integrating the findings from the qualitative and quantitative components of a study, called following a thread.[18] They state that this takes place at the analysis stage of the research process (figure). It begins with an initial analysis of each component to identify key themes and questions requiring further exploration. Then the researchers select a question or theme from one component and follow it across the other components—they call this the thread. The authors do not specify steps in this technique but offer a visual model for working between datasets. An approach similar to this has been undertaken in health services research, although the researchers did not label it as such, probably because the technique has not been used frequently in the literature (box)

Mixed methods matrix

A unique aspect of some mixed methods studies is the availability of both qualitative and quantitative data on the same cases. Data from the qualitative and quantitative components can be integrated at the analysis stage of a mixed methods study (figure). For example, in-depth interviews might be carried out with a sample of survey respondents, creating a subset of cases for which there is both a completed questionnaire and a transcript. Cases may be individuals, groups, organisations, or geographical areas.[9] All the data collected on a single case can be studied together, focusing attention on cases, rather than variables or themes, within a study. The data can be examined in detail for each case—for example, comparing people's responses to a questionnaire with their interview transcript. Alternatively, data on each case can be summarised and displayed in a matrix[8-20] along the lines of Miles and Huberman's meta-matrix.[21] Within a mixed methods matrix, the rows represent the cases for which there is both qualitative and quantitative data, and the columns display different data collected on each case. This allows researchers to pay attention to surprises and paradoxes between types of data on a single case and then look for patterns across all cases[20] in a qualitative cross case analysis.[21]

We used a mixed methods matrix to study the relation between types of team working and the extent of integration in mixed methods studies in health services research (table).[22] Quantitative data were extracted from the proposals, reports, and peer reviewed publications of 75 mixed methods studies, and these were analysed to describe the proportion of studies with integrated outputs

---

EXAMPLE OF FOLLOWING A THREAD[19]

amson and colleagues explored the effect of patient views on the appropriate use of services d help seeking using a survey of people registered at a general practice and semistructured erviews. The qualitative (22 interviews) and quantitative components (survey with 911 spondents) took place concurrently.

e researchers describe what they call an iterative or cyclical approach to analysis. Firstly, the eliminary findings from the interviews generated a hypothesis for testing in the survey data. A y theme from the interviews concerned the self rationing of services as a responsible way of ing scarce health care. This theme was then explored in the survey data by testing the hypothesis at people's views of the appropriate use of services would explain their help seeking behaviour. wever, there was no support for this hypothesis in the quantitative analysis because the half of rvey respondents who felt that health services were used inappropriately were as likely to report lp seeking for a series of symptoms presented in standardised vignettes as were respondents o thought that services were not used inappropriately. The researchers then followed the thread ck to the interview data to help interpret this finding.

er further analysis of the interview data the researchers understood that people considered the lp seeking of other people to be inappropriate, rather than their own. They also noted that feeling xious about symptoms was considered to be a good justification for seeking care. The researchers lowed this thread back into the survey data and tested whether anxiety levels about the mptoms in the standardised vignettes predicted help seeking behaviour. This second hypothesis s supported by the survey data. Following a thread led the researchers to conclude that patients o seek health care for seemingly minor problems have exceeded their thresholds for the trade-off tween not using services inappropriately and any anxiety caused by their symptoms.

---

e **Example of a mixed methods matrix for a study exploring the relationship between types eams and integration between qualitative and quantitative components of studies***[22]

dy	Evidence of integration in report†	Types of publications emerging‡	Qualitative expertise on the team	Team working	Respect for team members
	1	5	Yes	Close and friendly	Yes
	1	5	Yes	Single researcher	Yes
	1	4	No senior qualitative expertise on team but project researcher worked hard at it	Integrated team. The qualitative and quantitative researchers were in same department	Yes
	2	4	Yes. There was also expertise developing in mixed methods research	Integrated team. The lead researcher worked closely with qualitative and quantitative researchers	Initially some team members did not respect the qualitative research but learnt to as the study progressed
	2	4	Reported as no problem even though junior staff had no expertise	The junior researcher delivered both the qualitative and the quantitative components. The team was geographically close	Lead researcher did not respect the qualitative research but other senior team members did
	2	4	Yes, including mixed methods expertise	Worked well together. Lead researcher worked closely with qualitative and quantitative researchers	Yes

ws the first six cases and a selection of themes from the full matrix. The content of some of the original cells has changed to increase comprehension and protect confidentiality.
yes, 2=yes but more possible, 3=no.
one, 2=only qualitative, 3=only quantitative, 4=both published separately, 5=mixed methods article.

such as mixed methods journal articles. Two key variables in the quantitative component were whether the study was assessed as attempting to integrate qualitative or quantitative data or findings and the type of publications produced. We conducted qualitative interviews with 20 researchers who had worked on some of these studies to explore how mixed methods research was practised, including how the team worked together.

The shared cases between the qualitative and quantitative components were 21 mixed methods studies (because one interviewee had worked on two studies in the quantitative component). A matrix was formed with each of the 21 studies as a row. The first column of the matrix contained the study identification, the second column indicated whether integration had occurred in that project, and the third column the score for integration of publications emerging from the study. The rows were then ordered to show the most integrated cases first. This ordering of rows helped us to see patterns across rows.

The next columns were themes from the qualitative interview with a researcher from that project. For example, the first theme was about the expertise in qualitative research within the team and whether the interviewee reported this as adequate for the study. The matrix was then used in the context of the qualitative analysis to explore the issues that affected integration. In particular, it helped to identify negative cases (when someone in the analysis doesn't fit with the conclusions the analysis is coming to) within the qualitative analysis to facilitate understanding. Interviewees reported the need for experienced qualitative researchers on mixed methods studies to ensure that the qualitative component was published, yet two cases showed that this was neither necessary nor sufficient. This pushed us to explore other factors in a research team that helped generate outputs, and integrated outputs, from a mixed methods study.

Themes from a qualitative study can be summarised to the point where they are coded into quantitative data. In the matrix (table), the interviewee's perception of the adequacy of qualitative expertise on the team could have been coded as adequate=1 or not=2. This is called "quantitising" of qualitative data[23]; coded data can then be analysed with data from the quantitative component. This technique has been used to great effect in healthcare research to identify the discrepancy between health improvement assessed using quantitative measures and with in-depth interviews in a randomised controlled trial.[24]

Conclusion

We have presented three techniques for integration in mixed methods research in the hope that they will inspire researchers to explore what can be learnt from bringing together data from the qualitative and quantitative components of their studies. Using these techniques may give the process of integration credibility rather than leaving researchers feeling that they have "made things up." It may also encourage researchers to describe their approaches to integration, allowing them to be transparent and helping them to develop, critique, and improve on these techniques. Most importantly, we believe it may help researchers to generate further understanding from their research.

We have presented integration as unproblematic, but it is not. It may be easier for single researchers to use these techniques than a large research team. Large teams will need to pay attention to team dynamics, considering who will take responsibility for integration and who be taking part in the process. In addition, we have ta a technical stance here rather than paying attention different philosophical beliefs that may shape approac to integration. We consider that these techniques wc work in the context of a pragmatic or subtle realist sta adopted by some mixed methods researchers.[25] Finally is important to remember that these techniques are a to integration and are helpful only when applied v expertise.

Funding: Medical Research Council grant reference G106/1116

Competing interests: All authors have completed the unified competing interest form at www.icmje.org/coi_disclosure.pdf (available on request from the corresponding author) and declare financial support for the submitted work from the Medical Resear Council; no financial relationships with commercial entities that might have an interest in the submitted work; no spouses, partne or children with relationships with commercial entities that might have an interest in the submitted work; and no non-financial interests that may be relevant to the submitted work.

Contributors: AOC wrote the paper. JN and EM contributed to draft and all authors agreed the final version. AOC is guarantor.

Provenance and peer review: Not commissioned; externally peer reviewed.

1 Lingard L, Albert M, Levinson W. Grounded theory, mixed methods action research. BMJ 2008;337:a567.
2 Creswell JW, Fetters MD, Ivankova NV. Designing a mixed methods study in primary care. Ann Fam Med 2004;2:7-12.
3 Lewin S, Glenton C, Oxman AD. Use of qualitative methods alongsi randomised controlled trials of complex healthcare interventions: methodological study. BMJ 2009;339:b3496.
4 O'Cathain A, Murphy E, Nicholl J. Integration and publications as indicators of 'yield' from mixed methods studies. J Mix Methods F 2007;1:147-63.
5 Barbour RS. The case for combining qualitative and quantitative approaches in health services research. J Health Serv Res Policy 1999;4:39-43.
6 O'Cathain A, Nicholl J, Murphy E. Structural issues affecting mixed methods studies in health research: a qualitative study. BMC Med Methodol 2009;9:82.
7 Bryman A. Barriers to integrating quantitative and qualitative research. J Mix Methods Res 2007;1:8-22.
8 Creswell JW, Plano-Clark V. Designing and conducting mixed metho research . Sage, 2007.
9 Bazeley P. Analysing mixed methods data. In: Andrew S, Halcomb eds. Mixed methods research for nursing and the health sciences Wiley-Blackwell, 2009:84-118.
10 Sandelowski M. Triangles and crystals: on the geometry of qualita research. Res Nurs Health 1995;18:569-74.
11 Farmer T, Robinson K, Elliott SJ, Eyles J. Developing and implement a triangulation protocol for qualitative health research. Qual Healt Res 2006;16:377-94.
12 Foster RL. Addressing the epistemologic and practical issues in multimethod research: a procedure for conceptual triangulation. A Nurs Sci 1997;20:1-12.
13 Erzerberger C, Prein G. Triangulation: validity and empirically base hypothesis construction. Qual Quant 1997;31:141-54.
14 Fielding NG, Fielding JL. Linking data . Sage, 1986.
15 Moffatt S, White M, Mackintosh J, Howel D. Using quantitative and qualitative data in health services research—what happens when mixed method findings conflict? BMC Health Serv Res 2006;6:28.
16 Sampson FC, O'Cathain A, Goodacre S. Is primary angioplasty an acceptable alternative to thrombolysis? Quantitative and qualitativ study of patient and carer satisfaction. Health Expectations (forthcoming).
17 Morgan DL. Practical strategies for combining qualitative and quantitative methods: applications to health research. Qual Health Res 1998;8:362-76.
18 Moran-Ellis J, Alexander VD, Cronin A, Dickinson M, Fielding J, Sleney J, et al. Triangulation and integration: processes, claims and implications. Qualitative Research 2006;6:45-59.
19 Adamson J, Ben-Shlomo Y, Chaturvedi N, Donovan J. Exploring the impact of patient views on 'appropriate' use of services and help seeking: a mixed method study. Br J Gen Pract 2009;59:496-502.
20 Wendler MC. Triangulation using a meta-matrix. J Adv Nurs 2001;35:521-5.
21 Miles M, Huberman A. Qualitative data analysis: an expanded sourcebook . Sage, 1994.
22 O'Cathain A, Murphy E, Nicholl J. Multidisciplinary, interdisciplinary dysfunctional? Team working in mixed methods research. Qual Hea Res 2008;18:1574-85.
23 Sandelowski M. Combining qualitative and quantitative sampling, data collection, and analysis techniques in mixed-method studies. Res Nurs Health 2000;23:246-55.

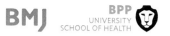

24 Campbell R, Quilty B, Dieppe P. Discrepancies between patients'
    assessments of outcome: qualitative study nested within a
    randomised controlled trial. *BMJ* 2003;326:252-3.
25 Mays N, Pope C. Assessing quality in qualitative research. *BMJ*
    2000;320:50-2.

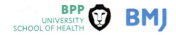

Dangers of non-specific composite outcome measures in clinical trials

David Prieto-Merino, lecturer[1], Liam Smeeth, professor[2], Tjeerd P van Staa, professor[2 3], Ian Roberts, professor[1]

[1]Clinical Trials Unit, London School of Hygiene and Tropical Medicine, London WC1E 7HT, UK

[2]Faculty of Epidemiology and Population Health, London School of Hygiene and Tropical Medicine

[3]Utrecht Institute for Pharmaceutical Sciences, Utrecht University, Utrecht, Netherlands

Correspondence to: D Prieto-Merino david.prieto@lshtm.ac.uk

Cite this as: BMJ 2013;347:f6782

DOI: 10.1136/bmj.f6782

http://www.bmj.com/content/347/bmj.f6782

According to international guidelines,[1] [2] outcome measures in a clinical trial should address the risks and benefits of a treatment, be relevant to patients, and be sufficiently common to make the trial feasible. In an attempt to meet these objectives many investigators select outcomes such as all cause mortality, all hospital admissions, or any adverse event. These outcomes can be thought of as composite outcomes as they combine multiple outcomes that are cause specific. All cause mortality is a popular outcome measure because it is believed to provide the net effect of the treatment, it seems more patient relevant than cause specific mortality, and it provides more outcomes so should increase statistical power. Another common approach to increase power is to use wide case definitions and sensitive tests.

In recent years several papers have reviewed and debated the use of composite outcomes in clinical trials.[3-9] Authors agree on their advantages and disadvantages, and a good summary can be found in a recent report from the European Network for Health Technology Assessment.[10] Briefly, the main objection to the use of composite outcomes is that, if the treatment has different effects on the different components of the outcome, the net effect on the composite outcome is difficult to interpret. It also complicates patient management decisions, raising the question of which particular component outcome is more relevant for each patient.

However, in the ongoing debate little emphasis has been given to the fact that, by including events that are not causally related to the treatment (either by using a composite outcome or by misclassifying events with a wide case definition), the overall effect of the trial will be diluted towards the null. In this paper we explain why dilution occurs, provide examples of trials where this has happened, and discuss how dilution can offset many of the supposed advantages.

Motivating example: planning a clinical trial

Having reviewed the existing evidence, you believe that β blockers might improve lung function and so reduce hospital admissions in patients with chronic obstructive pulmonary disease (COPD), although you are worried that they might cause severe bronchospasm in some patients. You decide to conduct a randomised controlled trial comparing β blockers

ABSTRACT

Composite outcomes seem an attractive method to increase statistical power, but they can mask the effect of treatment

with placebo in people with moderate COPD. Because the large burden on health services and the importance ■ the patients, you define the primary outcome as the ri of hospital admission over one year. Your practice recor show that patients with moderate COPD have a 40% risk ■ being admitted to hospital each year (although only h of admissions are for COPD). The statistician says that study of about 1510 patients followed up for a year shou have enough power to detect a 20% decrease in admissio (that is, from 40% to 32%). Because of your concern abo bronchospasm, participants are asked to keep a dia of episodes of wheeze or shortness of breath as well more severe symptoms. Severe bronchospasm is rare people with COPD (about one episode per 10 person year although many feel wheezy or short of breath (about on a week).

Imagine that trial recruitment went well and that tab 1 shows the (hypothetical) results. There is no significa reduction in hospital admissions and no evidence increase in the adverse event. Should you conclude that blockers have no beneficial or adverse effects?

This example has been made up to show how re treatment effects can be diluted by using non-speci outcome measures. Patients are admitted to hospital f many different reasons. "Any hospital admission" c be considered a composite of different cause speci admissions. In this example, half of admissions were relate to COPD. If we examine only COPD related admissions the is some evidence of a treatment effect. We see the sam thing with adverse events. Even though β blockers d increase the risk of severe bronchospasm, the ability the trial to detect this effect is lost altogether because t outcome measure includes wheeze and shortness of breat which are common in COPD patients and are not affected ■ the intervention. If outcomes that are causally related to t trial treatment are combined with those that are not, t estimate of the treatment effect is diluted towards the n and we may fail to identify potentially important benefi or harms.

Explaining treatment effects with a causal mechanism model

The effect of a treatment on a health outcome can be show using the causal mechanism model described by Rothma and colleagues.[11] For a patient to experience a specifi health outcome, a particular set of events, conditions, characteristics must occur. This set is called the caus mechanism. The causal mechanism is considered sufficie to produce the health outcome, and each compone cause is necessary in the sense that had it been absen

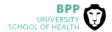

Results for an example trial of β blockers in chronic obstructive pulmonary disease (COPD)

Outcome	β blocker (n=775)* No of patients/ events	β blocker (n=775)* Risk/rate†	Control (n=755)* No of patients/ events	Control (n=755)* Risk/rate†	Relative risk/rate† (95% CI)	P value
spital admission						
cause	272	0.35	302	0.4	0.90 (0.79 to 1.02)	<0.12
PD related	121	0.16	151	0.2	0.80 (0.65 to 0.99)	<0.045
verse events						
shortness of ath	39 746	0.1442	39 444	0.1431	1.01 (0.99 to 1.02)	<0.29
ere nchospasm	378	0.0014	76	0.0003	4.96 (3.91 to 6.40)	<0.0001

575 patient days of follow-up.
*pital admissions are described as risks and adverse events as rates.

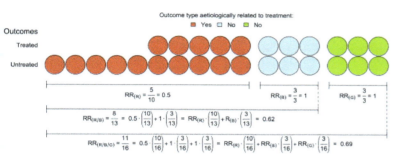

Example of composite outcome, only one part of which (red outcome) is related to treatment. We me the same number of patients in each arm of the trial. (RR= relative risk, R=red, B=blue, and een)

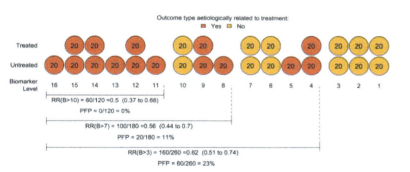

Example of misclassification of outcomes in a randomised controlled trial based on biomarker , 20 patients per circle and assuming a total of 2000 patients randomised to each arm. The effect eatment on aetiologically related outcomes (red circles) is relative risk=0.5. (RR= relative risk, omarker, PFP=proportion of false positive results)

this example, the red outcome is causally related to the treatment whereas the blue and green outcomes are not.

Composite outcomes

A composite outcome combines different outcomes (with different causal mechanisms).[1] The effect of a treatment on a composite outcome is a weighted average of its effects on the outcomes that are combined. In fig 1 the treatment halves the occurrence of the red outcome (relative risk =0.5) but has no effect on the blue outcome (relative risk=1.0). The relative risk of the outcome red or blue is the weighted average of the relative risks for the red and blue outcomes: relative risk red or blue=0.5(10/13)+1.0(3/13). Where (10/13) and (3/13) are the relative weights of the red and the blue outcomes in the untreated group. If a composite includes outcomes that are not causally related to the treatment, the relative risk for the composite is diluted towards the null.[12] Because few treatments will be causally related to all causes of death, all cause mortality is a composite outcome that combines causally related causes of death with those unrelated to the treatment.

Misclassification of outcome

Many trials use diagnostic tests to assess the presence or absence of a health outcome. For example, troponin levels might be used to determine the presence or absence of a myocardial infarction.[13] Whatever method is used to assess outcome, there will be false positives and false negative results. The number of false positives divided by the total number of positive outcomes is the proportion of false positives. Figure 2 shows the effect of outcome misclassification on the relative risk in a trial. Each arm is assumed to have 2000 participants and each circle represents 20 outcomes. The treatment effect estimated using the causally related outcome is 100/200 (relative risk=0.50, 95% confidence interval 0.40 to 0.63). Some related outcomes have low biomarker values and some unrelated outcomes have high biomarker values. The misclassification of outcomes, the proportion of false positives, and the relative risk will change depending on the biomarker's cut-off value. If we define the outcome as present when the biomarker value is more than seven, we will miss 20 causally related outcomes in the treatment group and 40 in the untreated group. We also add 20 false positive outcomes to both groups. Because false positive outcomes are included, the relative risk moves closer to the null (relative risk=0.56, 0.44 to 0.70). The dilution is greater if we define the outcome as present when the biomarker value is more than three, because there are even more false positive results (0.62, 0.51 to 0.74). Rodgers and McMahon[14] showed that, whatever the true relative risk, the estimated relative risk moves towards the null as the proportion of false positive results increases.

Figure 2 also shows that as the number of outcomes increases, the precision of the relative risk increases (narrower confidence interval). However, in this case we are more certain about the answer to a different question. With the biomarker cut-off at 3, we have a precise estimate (0.62, 0.51 to 0.74) but one that excludes the true relative risk of 0.5. Notice that, on the other hand, the higher the value required in the biomarker, the more real outcomes that we will fail to detect (false negative results). The increase in

that outcome would not have occurred. The same health outcome might result from different causal mechanisms sharing some component causes, and different outcomes might arise from similar causal mechanisms. A trial treatment has the potential to cause a change in health outcome by blocking (or adding) one or more of the necessary component causes in the causal mechanism. We would say that a health outcome is causally related to a treatment if some causal mechanisms contain component causes that are blocked by the treatment. Figure 1 shows a hypothetical trial with three outcomes: red, blue, and green. For simplicity, we assume that the same number of patients was allocated to the treated and untreated groups, so that the relative risk is the ratio of patient outcomes. Treatment can prevent some (but not all) of the red outcome. In

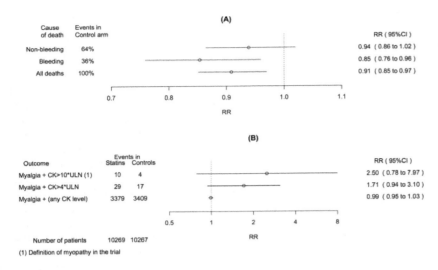

Fig 3 Examples of composite outcomes diluting effects of treatment from (*a*) the CRASH-2 trial[15] and (*b*) the Heart Protection Study[16] (CK=creatine kinase, ULN=upper limit of normal)

false negative results will reduce the power of the analysis but will not cause dilution as this is only caused by the inclusion of false positives.

Examples from real trials

The CRASH-2 trial is a randomised placebo controlled trial of tranexamic acid versus placebo in bleeding trauma patients.[15] The primary outcome was "all-cause mortality in hospital within 4 weeks of injury." However, tranexamic acid was expected to work by reducing bleeding in which case death from bleeding is arguably the causally related outcome. The relative risk for death from bleeding with tranexamic acid was 0.85 whereas the relative risk for non-bleeding deaths was 0.94. In the untreated group, 36% of deaths were due to bleeding and 64% to other causes. The relative risk on all cause mortality was the weighted average of the two effects: relative risk=0.91=0.85×0.36 + 0.94×0.64 (fig 3(*a*)).

The Heart Protection Study is a randomised controlled trial of simvastatin versus placebo in 20 500 patients at high risk of cardiovascular events.[16] The aim was to evaluate effects of cholesterol lowering on patient outcomes. There were concerns about a possible increase in the risk of myopathy, defined as "unexplained muscle pains or weakness" (myalgia) with raised levels of the enzyme creatine kinase. Reports of myalgia were collected from trial participants and creatine kinase was measured in these patients. Figure 3(*b*) shows the effect of simvastatin on myalgia for different cut-off values of creatine kinase. As the cut-off value is reduced there are more myalgia outcomes and so the confidence interval is narrower. However, the relative risk moves closer to the null. Myalgia is a common symptom and is likely to have many different mechanisms. Most cases will not be causally related to the treatment. Nevertheless, the possibility that some cases might be related to treatment cannot be excluded from these data.

Discussion

Composite outcomes are often used to obtain more outcome events and thus increase statistical power.[17] This is reasonable if all components of the composite are causally relevant and the treatment effects are similar. If the treatment effects vary considerably between outcome components the trial provides a more precise answer but to an irrelevant average effect that does not represent any

meaningful clinical effect. Furthermore, if some compone are not causally related to the treatment, the effec treatment will be diluted towards the null, offsetting gain in precision and not increasing the power of the (as shown in the examples above). The real solution may to increase the sample size until there is enough powe answer the question for the outcome of interest.

The CONSORT guideline recommends that the m outcome should be something "relevant to the patien It is tempting to assume that composites such as cause mortality, any hospital admission, overall qua of life, or any adverse event, might be more relevan patients than a particular cause of death or a partic adverse effect. However, such composite outcomes may provide the information needed for patient care. In pract each patient has a different risk profile for each of components of the composite. Even if all cause morta is the outcome that matters to patients, knowing how treatment affects specific causes of death is more impor for patient management.

It is also tempting to believe that all cause morta provides the net effect of the treatment[17] and so provides attractive summary for policy makers. However, conclusi made on the basis of the effect on a composite outco are applicable to the population where the trial took p and are not readily generalisable to other populations.[10] net effect on a composite outcome in a given populat depends on the relative frequency of the compon outcomes. Even if the effects on specific compon outcomes are the same across populations, the net ef on the composite will not be the same if the distribu of component outcomes varies. In particular, the net ef of the composite outcome will be diluted in populati where the components that are not causally related to treatment were common. In a multisite or multinatic trial, the net effect might vary by hospital or country eve the specific effects remain constant.

In clinical practice, doctors often prefer highly sensi diagnostic tests that have a low proportion of false nega results to ensure that few patients are denied an effec treatment. However, in clinical trials, it is important to highly specific diagnostic tests that have a low propor of false positive results to prevent dilution of the treatm effect.

Contributors: DP-M and IR did the main writing and LS and TvS ma the corrections. All authors critically revised the draft for importar intellectual content, and gave final approval of the version to be published. DP-M is the guarantor for the study.

Competing interests: All authors read and understood the BMJ pol on declaration of interests and have no relevant interests to decla

Provenance and peer review: Not commissioned; externally peer reviewed.

1 ICH Expert Working Group. Statistical principles for clinical trials E9 International conference on harmonisation of technical requireme for registration of pharmaceuticals for human use. 1998. Technical report. www.ich.org/products/guidelines/efficacy/efficacy-single/ article/statistical-principles-for-clinical-trials.html. Accessed 26-Sept-2013.
2 Moher D, Hopewell S, Schulz KF, Montori V, Gotzsche PC, Devereau et al. CONSORT 2010 explanation and elaboration: updated guidelir for reporting parallel group randomised trials. *BMJ* 2010;340:c869.
3 Cordoba G, Schwartz L, Woloshin S, Bae H, Gotzsche PC. Definition, reporting, and interpretation of composite outcomes in clinical tri systematic review. *BMJ* 2010;341:c3920.
4 Ferreira-Gonzalez I, Busse JW, Heels-Ansdell D, Montori VM, Akl EA, Bryant DM, et al. Problems with use of composite end points in cardiovascular trials: systematic review of randomised controlled trials. *BMJ* 2007;334:786.
5 Ferreira-Gonzalez I, Permanyer-Miralda G, Busse JW, Bryant DM, Montori VM, Alonso-Coello P, et al. Composite endpoints in clinical trials: the trees and the forest. *J Clin Epidemiol* 2007;60:660-1.

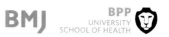

6   Ferreira-Gonzalez I, Permanyer-Miralda G, Busse JW, Bryant DM, Montori VM, Alonso-Coello P, et al. Methodologic discussions for using and interpreting composite endpoints are limited, but still identify major concerns. *J Clin Epidemiol* 2007;60:651-7, discussion 658-62.

7   Freemantle N, Calvert M, Wood J, Eastaugh J, Griffin C. Composite outcomes in randomized trials greater precision but with greater uncertainty? *JAMA* 2003;289:2554-9.

8   Freemantle N, Calvert M. Weighing the pros and cons for composite outcomes in clinical trials. *J Clin Epidemiol* 2007;60:658-9.

9   Montori VM, Permanyer-Miralda G, Ferreira-Gonzalez I, Busse JW, Pacheco-Huergo V, Bryant D, et al. Validity of composite end points in clinical trials. *BMJ* 2005;330:594-6.

10   European Network for Health Technology Assessment. Endpoints used for REA of pharmaceuticals: composite endpoints. 2013. www.eunethta.eu/outputs/ methodological-guideline-rea-pharmaceuticals-composite-endpoints.

11   Rothman KJ, Lash TL, Greenland S. Modern epidemiology. Lippincott Williams and Wilkins, 2012.

12   Kessler KM. Combining composite endpoints: counterintuitive or a mathematical impossibility? *Circulation* 2003;107:e70.

13   Cockburn J, Behan M, de Belder A, Clayton T, Stables R, Oldroyd K, et al. Use of troponin to diagnose periprocedural myocardial infarction: effect on composite endpoints in the British Bifurcation Coronary Study (BBC ONE). *Heart* 2012;98:1431-5.

14   Rodgers A, McMahon S. Systematic underestimation of treatment effects as a result of diagnostic test inaccuracy: implications for the interpretation and design of thromboprophylaxis trials. *Thromb Haemost* 1995;73:167-71.

15   CRASH-2 Collaborators. Effects of tranexamic acid on death, vascular occlusive events, and blood transfusion in trauma patients with significant haemorrhage (CRASH-2): a randomised, placebo-controlled trial. *Lancet* 2010;376:1-10.

16   HPS Collaborative Group. MRC/BHF Heart Protection Study of cholesterol lowering with simvastatin in 20,536 high-risk individuals: a randomised placebo-controlled trial. *Lancet* 2002;360:7-22.

17   Lubsen J, Kirwan B. Combined endpoints: can we use them? *Stat Med* 2002;21:2959-70.

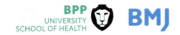

Cascade diagrams for depicting complex interventions in randomised trials

Richard Hooper, senior lecturer in medical statistics[1], Robert J Froud, senior research fellow, clinical trials[2] [3], Stephen A Bremner, lecturer in medical statistics[1], Rafael Perera, university lecturer in medical statistics[4], Sandra Eldridge, professor of biostatistics[1]

[1]Centre for Primary Care and Public Health, Blizard Institute, Queen Mary University of London, London E1 2AT, UK

[2]Clinical Trials Unit, Division of Health Sciences, University of Warwick, Warwick, UK

[3]Norges Helsehoyskole, Campus Kristiania, Norway

[4]Centre for Evidence Based Medicine, Department of Primary Health Care, University of Oxford, Oxford, UK

Correspondence to: R Hooper
r.l.hooper@qmul.ac.uk

Cite this as: *BMJ* 2013;347:f6681

DOI: 10.1136/bmj.f6681

http://www.bmj.com/content/347/bmj.f6681

Many medical interventions—particularly non-pharmacological ones—are complex, consisting of multiple interacting components targeted at different organisational levels.[1] [2] Published descriptions of complex interventions often do not contain enough detail to enable their replication.[2] [3] [4] [5] Reports of behaviour change interventions should include descriptions of setting, mode, intensity, and duration, and characteristics of the participants.[6] Graphical methods, such as that showing the relative timing of assessments and intervention components,[7] may improve clarity of reporting. However, these approaches do not reveal the connections between the different "actors" in a complex intervention.[8] Different audiences may want different things from a description of an intervention, but visualising relationships between actors can clarify crucial features such as the fidelity with which the intervention is passed down a chain of actors[9] and possible routes of contamination between treatment arms. Here we describe a new graphical approach—the cascade diagram—that highlights these potential problems.

Hierarchical interventions

Figure 1a is a schematic illustration of a hierarchically delivered intervention. At the top is a health professional or primary investigator who trains several health professionals at the next level down to deliver the intervention to a common standard. Each of these second level professionals then delivers the intervention to patients at the third level. In this example we suppose that patients are treated in groups: thus each patient receives input from a health professional (the arrow coming down from the second level) and also from the other patients in their group (drawn as a circulating arrow at the lowest level), and these inputs combine or interact to produce a health benefit.

In fig 1b we have uncluttered the diagram by separating out the information showing the relationships between actors at different levels. The circulating arrow allows us to show the contact between patients and the level at which it occurs without having to depict more than one patient. We can no longer see how many actors there are at different levels, or the range of their characteristics: these things are important to report, but current guidelines recommend that they be included in the CONSORT flowchart and in text or tables.[6] [10] What we are left with is a diagram showing the flow from the source of the intervention, at the top, down to the patient who receives it, at the bottom. This simple idea is the basis for the cascade diagram.

Figure 2a shows the graphical elements that make up a cascade diagram: actors (rectangular boxes), hierarchical levels not represented by an actor (rounded boxes), and intervention components (arrows with labels, indexed in a separate key). As an example we illustrate in fig 2b a parenting intervention for preterm infants described by

ABSTRACT

Clarity about how trial interventions are delivered is important for researchers and those who might want to use their results. A new graphical representation aims to help make complex interventions clearer

Johnson and colleagues.[11] In this study the trial manag trained research nurses in the delivery of the acti intervention, and each nurse delivered the intervention mothers of babies in neonatal intensive care units. Mothe then cared for their infants, whose cognitive outcomes we assessed at 2 years.

As a general rule, our diagrams exclude actors who provi only routine care, with no influence from any experiment intervention. In fig 2 we have excluded intensive care u staff, who were not trained in the intervention. We hav however, included the neonatal intensive care units the hierarchy because it allows us to show the extent communication between mothers taking part in the stud The exchange of information between mothers is show as a circulating arrow extending back as far (horizontal as the level of the intensive care unit and no further, t assumption being that contact between mothers exten only as far as those attending the same unit, and not, f example, to those seen by the same research nurse.

The diagonal arrangement of actors denotes the casca of an intervention through a hierarchy. Different acto at the same level, who do not stand in a hierarchical sequential relationship to each other, can be shown o under the other, or side by side, depending on what wor best in the diagram. We use singular rather than plu nouns in our actor boxes ("research nurse" rather th "research nurses") to avoid ambiguity about who delive the intervention. A box may contain more than one pers if they interact jointly with the actor at the next level—f example, we might write "general practitioner and practi nurse" or simply "practice staff" if these were the people patient had contact with—but we would recommend writir for example, "midwife" rather than "midwives" unless ea participant was seen by a whole team of midwives.

Trials

So far we have discussed how to illustrate the delivery an active intervention, but we would like our diagrams go further and show the different treatment arms in a tri In fig 3 we illustrate our suggested approach using a varie of simple two arm trial designs.

Figure 3a shows the simplest kind of trial, with participa randomised individually. We indicate randomisation wi a shaded banner running behind the two randomis groups. As before, we do not include actors who provi only routine care. In this example, the control participa

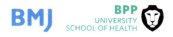

is isolated graphically: there is no link through which he or she can receive the active intervention—that is, no possible route for contamination.

Figure 3b shows how an individually randomised design can lead to contamination in something like a general practice setting, where patients attending the same practice share information about the care they receive. Practice is shown as an organisational marker, with no actors at this level involved in delivering the intervention. Patient to patient contact within a practice is indicated by the circulating arrow, which shows information circulating within the bounds defined by a practice. Because there are control and intervention participants at the same practice, this circulating flow provides a route through which the active intervention can pass to, or contaminate, control participants.

Figure 3c shows how a cluster randomised trial avoids contamination in this situation.[12] If we assume that the flow of information between participants does not extend between clusters—in this case between patients at different general practices—then the circulating flow among control

participants is effectively isolated from the flow among intervention participants. The diagram shows that there is no route through which the active intervention can pass to control participants.

Finally, fig 3d shows a cluster randomised trial in which the intervention is aimed at cluster (practice) level, its effects then being cascaded down to individual participants. Again, contamination is avoided by randomising in clusters.

More complex interventions

We developed cascade diagrams after considering how to describe real life trials of complex interventions. Here we illustrate one example, the Older People's Exercise Intervention in Residential and Nursing Accommodation (OPERA) trial,[13] which was a trial of an exercise programme to reduce depression. We consulted in depth on the graphical representation of OPERA with its chief investigators as well as those conducting a process evaluation of the trial, to produce summaries that they found helpful. The results are shown in the web appendix, where we present the cascade diagram, the diagram proposed by Perera and colleagues (the PaT plot),[14] and the CONSORT flowchart for OPERA, to show how these approaches complement each other (the numbers in the CONSORT flowchart have been left blank, as these were unpublished at the time we developed the supplement).

The CONSORT flowchart, which should always be included in a trial report,[10] summarises the flow of individuals through a trial, whereas the cascade diagram is a model of the flow of interventions. The PaT plot describes the timing of different intervention components, while the cascade diagram shows the relationships between the actors delivering them. Detailed information about intervention components is included in the key to the cascade diagram, which also acts as the key to the PaT plot. Between them, the cascade diagram, PaT plot, key, and CONSORT flowchart form a complete description of a trial of a multicomponent, multilevel intervention such as OPERA.

Even for a complex intervention, we suggest that the cascade diagram be kept as simple as possible. Actors who only provide routine care can be left out unless that care is contaminated by an experimental intervention, though we will always need to show, at the lowest level, the individual participant or unit of analysis. Different boxes referring to the same type of actor are needed when different actors are randomised into different arms; when the same actor fulfils more than one role in a trial, however, there should just be one box for that actor. The appearance of more than one of the same kind of actor in the diagram, unless at the randomisation level, alerts us to situations where actors are separated into non-randomised groups—for example, midwives at a maternity unit being divided non-randomly into those who treat intervention mothers and those who treat controls—a situation that should usually be avoided.

Discussion

We have introduced a simple but powerful graphical approach to describe the delivery of a complex intervention in a trial. The method focuses on aspects that are not well addressed by existing approaches to reporting.

A recent, evidence based assessment of the key dimensions in describing complex interventions distinguished between the timing of intervention components, for which a diagrammatic approach has already been successfully introduced,[7] and other features— including "structure and

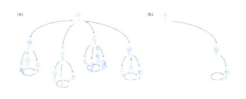

Fig 1 (*a*) Illustration of a hierarchically delivered intervention: a health professional or primary investigator at the top level trains several health professionals to deliver the intervention to a common standard; each second level professional then delivers the intervention to patients in a group setting. Circulating arrows show the intervention circulating within a group (the second level professionals are trained separately and independently, so there is no circulating arrow at this level). (*b*) Abstraction of the first diagram showing the relationships between actors at different levels

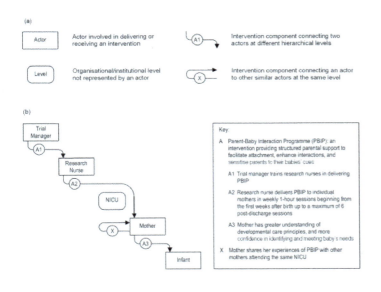

2 (*a*) Graphical elements making up the cascade diagram. (*b*) Cascade diagram for the parent-baby interaction programme (PBIP), a parenting intervention for very preterm infants in neonatal intensive care units (NICU)[11]

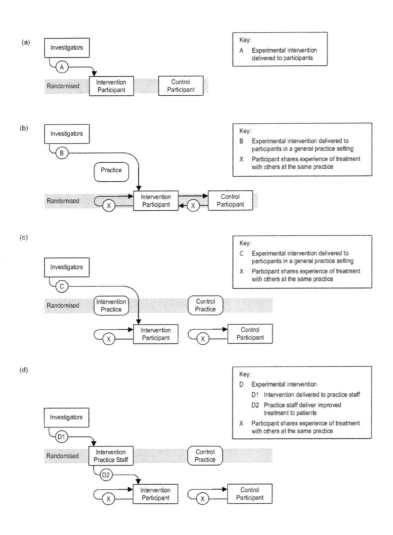

Fig 3 Cascade diagrams for various designs of randomised controlled trial: (*a*) a trial with individuals randomised to two arms; (*b*) an individually randomised trial in a general practice setting, showing contamination; (*c*) the same trial cluster randomised by practice; (*d*) a cluster randomised trial of an intervention delivered by general practice staff

altered by circulating currents within hierarchical levels. box representing each actor in the diagram is a "black b arrows enter and leave but may combine inside the bo non-linear ways.

We have limited the range of graphical elements the diagrams to make them as intuitive as possible, researchers may want to play with them further example, different arrow styles could distinguish interven components according to whether the standardisation be proposed was by function or form.[15 18]

Graphical methods in general continue to inte researchers.[18 19] Graphs and figures can be included online extras in a journal article even when editorial po limits the number of figures in the print version. Casc diagrams have some features in common with Uni Modelling Language (UML) sequence diagrams, wh are also beginning to find applications in health serv research.[20] A Microsoft Word toolkit for producing casc diagrams is available from the authors.

Commentators agree that much needs to be done improve the reporting of trials of complex interventio [3 4 5 6] The more people are able to understand what ot researchers have done, the more likely they are to reprodu cite, and discuss this work. We offer our diagramm approach as one new tool to aid in this complex task.

We thank Martin Underwood and Stephanie Taylor, chief investigat of the OPERA trial, and David Ellard, who conducted a process evaluation of OPERA, for their input into the OPERA example. We a thank the reviewers of earlier manuscripts for helpful comments.

Contributors: RH conceived the graphical approach following a cou on cluster randomised trials given by SE. The authors developed t method in consultation with clinical trialists, applying the method real examples and revising it in the light of feedback from trialists reviewers, and others. RH led on writing the manuscript, and all authors contributed to the final version. RH is the guarantor.

Competing interests: We have read and understood the BMJ Group policy on declaration of interests and have no relevant interests t declare.

Provenance and peer review: Not commissioned; externally peer reviewed.

1   Campbell M, Fitzpatrick R, Haines A, Kinmonth AL, Sandercock P, Spiegelhalter D, et al. Framework for design and evaluation of complex interventions to improve health. *BMJ* 2000;321:694-6.
2   Craig P, Dieppe P, Macintyre S, Michie S, Nazareth I, Petticrew M. Developing and evaluating complex interventions: the new Medica Research Council guidance. *BMJ* 2008;337:a1655.
3   Pino C, Boutron I, Ravaud P. Inadequate description of educational interventions in ongoing randomized controlled trials. *Trials* 2012;13:63.
4   Michie S, Fixsen D, Grimshaw JM, Eccles MP. Specifying and report complex behaviour change interventions: the need for a scientific method. *Implement Sci* 2009;4:40.
5   Glasziou P, Meats E, Heneghan C, Shepperd S. What is missing from descriptions of treatment in trials and reviews? *BMJ* 2008;336:1472
6   Abraham C. WIDER recommendations. 2013. www.interventiondesi co.uk/?page_id=9.
7   Perera R, Heneghan C, Yudkin P. Graphical method for depicting randomised trials of complex interventions. *BMJ* 2007;334:127-9.
8   Glasziou P, Chalmers I, Altman DG, Bastian H, Boutron I, Brice A, et al. Taking healthcare interventions from trial to practice. *BMJ* 2010;341:c3852.
9   Bellg AJ, Borrelli B, Resnick B, Hecht J, Minicucci DS, Ory M, et al. Enhancing treatment fidelity in health behavior change studies: best practices and recommendations from the NIH Behavior Chang Consortium. *Health Psychol* 2004;23:443-51.
10   Boutron I, Moher D, Altman DG, Schulz KF, Ravaud P. Extending the CONSORT statement to randomized trials of nonpharmacologic treatment: explanation and elaboration. *Ann Intern Med* 2008;148:295-309.
11   Johnson S, Whitelaw A, Glazebrook C, Israel C, Turner R, White IR, et al. Randomized trial of a parenting intervention for very preterm infants: outcome at 2 years. *J Pediatr* 2009;155:488-94.
12   Donner A, Klar, N. Cluster randomization trials. *Stat Method Med R* 2000;9:2.
13   Underwood M, Eldridge S, Lamb S, Potter R, Sheehan B, Slowther AM, et al. The OPERA trial: protocol for a randomised trial of an exercise intervention for older people in residential and nursing accommodation. *Trials* 2011;12:27.

architecture" and dependence on healthcare professionals—which our cascade diagrams attempt to depict.[15] Cascade diagrams may be useful after a study as a tool facilitating implementation or evidence synthesis, and before a study to encourage researchers to reflect on their design.[4 8] Managers considering how to adopt a published intervention can use the diagram to compare their institutional context with the one in which the intervention was evaluated.[15] At the design stage researchers can show design choices and identify methodological problems such as contamination or non-randomised groups—part of the crucial "modelling" phase in the development and evaluation of a complex intervention.[16] Contamination arising through contact between individuals at one level of a hierarchy is not always a bad thing: at the level of individual participants it can help to reinforce an intervention; at an intermediate health professional level it can help to standardise it.

Cascade diagrams are particularly useful for describing interventions delivered in a hierarchical context and for those whose complexity arises from a truly complex system, not just a complicated one.[17] For example, the diagram shows how, rather than flowing straight down a cascading sequence of actors, an intervention can be reinforced or

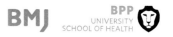

14 Perera R, Heneghan C, Yudkin, P. PaT plot. 2013. www.cebm.net/index.aspx?o=4200.

15 Wells M, Williams B, Treweek S, Coyle J, Taylor J. Intervention description is not enough: evidence from an in-depth multiple case study on the untold role and impact of context in randomised controlled trials of seven complex interventions. *Trials* 2012;13:95.

16 UK Medical Research Council. Complex interventions guidance. 2008. www.mrc.ac.uk/complexinterventionsguidance.

17 Shiell A, Hawe P, Gold L. Complex interventions or complex systems? Implications for health economic evaluation. *BMJ* 2008;336:1281-3.

18 Hawe P, Shiell A, Riley T. Complex interventions: how "out of control" can a randomised controlled trial be? *BMJ* 2004;328:1561-3.

19 Pitt M, Stahl-Timmins W, Anderson R, Stein K. Using information graphics in health technology assessment: toward a structured approach. *Int J Technol Assess Health Care* 2009;25:555-63.

20 Kumarapeli P, de Lusignan S, Koczan P, Jones B, Sheeler I. The feasibility of using UML to compare the impact of different brands of computer system on the clinical consultation. *Inform Primary Care* 2007;15:245-5.

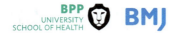

Recommendations for examining and interpreting funnel plot asymmetry in meta-analyses of randomised controlled trials

Jonathan A C Sterne, professor[1], Alex J Sutton, professor[2], John P A Ioannidis, professor and director[3], Norma Terrin, associate professor[4], David R Jones, professor[2], Joseph Lau, professor[4], James Carpenter, reader[5], Gerta Rücker, research assistant[6], Roger M Harbord, research associate[1], Christopher H Schmid, professor[4], Jennifer Tetzlaff, research coordinator[7], Jonathan J Deeks, professor[8], Jaime Peters, research fellow[9], Petra Macaskill, associate professor[10], Guido Schwarzer, research assistant[6], Sue Duval, assistant professor[11], Douglas G Altman, professor[12], David Moher, senior scientist[7], Julian P T Higgins, senior statistician[13]

[1]School of Social and Community Medicine, University of Bristol, Bristol BS8 2PS, UK

[2]Department of Health Sciences, University of Leicester, Leicester, UK

Correspondence to: J A C Sterne jonathan.sterne@bristol.ac.uk

[4]Institute for Clinical Research and Health Policy Studies, Tufts Medical Center, Boston, MA, USA

[5]Medical Statistics Unit, London School of Hygiene and Tropical Medicine, London, UK

[6]Institute of Medical Biometry and Medical Informatics, University Medical Center Freiburg, Germany

[7]Clinical Epidemiology Program, Ottawa Hospital Research Institute, Ottawa, Ontario, Canada

[8]School of Health and Population Sciences, University of Birmingham, Birmingham, UK

[9]Peninsula Medical School, University of Exeter, Exeter, UK

[10]School of Public Health, University of Sydney, NSW, Australia

[11]University of Minnesota School of Public Health, Minneapolis, MN, USA

[12]Centre for Statistics in Medicine, University of Oxford, Oxford, UK

[13]MRC Biostatistics Unit, Cambridge, UK

Cite this as: BMJ 2011;342:d4002

DOI: 10.1136/bmj.d4002

http://www.bmj.com/content/343/bmj.d4002

The 1997 paper describing the test for funnel plot asymmetry proposed by Egger et al [1] is one of the most cited articles in the history of BMJ.[1] Despite the recommendations contained in this and subsequent papers,[2][3] funnel plot asymmetry is often, wrongly, equated with publication or other reporting biases. The use and appropriate interpretation of funnel plots and tests for funnel plot asymmetry have been controversial because of questions about statistical validity,[4] disputes over appropriate interpretation,[3][5][6] and low power of the tests.[2]

This article recommends how to examine and interpret funnel plot asymmetry (also known as small study effects[2]) in meta-analyses of randomised controlled trials. The recommendations are based on a detailed MEDLINE review of literature published up to 2007 and discussions among methodologists, who extended and adapted guidance previously summarised in the Cochrane Handbook for Systematic Reviews of Interventions.[7]

What is a funnel plot?

A funnel plot is a scatter plot of the effect estimates from individual studies against some measure of each study's size or precision. The standard error of the effect estimate is often chosen as the measure of study size and plotted on the vertical axis[8] with a reversed scale that places the larger, most powerful studies towards the top. The effect estimates from smaller studies should scatter more widely at the bottom, with the spread narrowing among larger studies.[9]

ABSTRACT

Funnel plots, and tests for funnel plot asymmetry, have been widely used to examine bias in the results of meta-analyses. Funnel plot asymmetry should not be equated with publication bias, because it has a number of other possible causes. This article describes how to interpret funnel plot asymmetry, recommends appropriate tests, and explains the implications for choice of meta-analysis model

In the absence of bias and between study heterogenei the scatter will be due to sampling variation alone and t plot will resemble a symmetrical inverted funnel (fig 1). triangle centred on a fixed effect summary estimate a extending 1.96 standard errors either side will include abo 95% of studies if no bias is present and the fixed effe assumption (that the true treatment effect is the same each study) is valid. The appendix on bmj.com discuss choice of axis in funnel plots.

Implications of heterogeneity, reporting bias, and chance

Heterogeneity, reporting bias, and chance may all lead asymmetry or other shapes in funnel plots (box). Funn plot asymmetry may also be an artefact of the choice statistics being plotted (see appendix). The presence of a shape in a funnel plot is contingent on the studies havi a range of standard errors, since otherwise they would on a horizontal line.

Heterogeneity

Statistical heterogeneity refers to differences betwee study results beyond those attributable to chance. It ma arise because of clinical differences between studies (f example, setting, types of participants, or implementatio of the intervention) or methodological differences (su as extent of control over bias). A random effects model often used to incorporate heterogeneity in meta-analyse If the heterogeneity fits with the assumptions of th model, a funnel plot will be symmetrical but with addition horizontal scatter. If heterogeneity is large it may overwhel the sampling error, so that the plot appears cylindrical.

Heterogeneity will lead to funnel plot asymmetry if it induces a correlation between study sizes and interventio effects.[5] For example, substantial benefit may be see

SUMMARY POINTS

- Inferences on the presence of bias or heterogeneity should consider different causes of funnel plot asymmetry and should not be based on visual inspection of funnel plots alone
- They should be informed by contextual factors, including the plausibility of publication bias as an explanation for the asymmetry
- Testing for funnel plot asymmetry should follow the recommendations detailed in this article
- The fixed and random effects estimates of the intervention effect should be compared when funnel plot asymmetry exists in a meta-analysis with between study heterogeneity

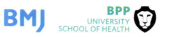

only in high risk patients, and these may be preferentially included in early, small studies.[10] Or the intervention may have been implemented less thoroughly in larger studies, resulting in smaller effect estimates compared with smaller studies.[11]

Figure 2 shows funnel plot asymmetry arising from heterogeneity that is due entirely to there being three distinct subgroups of studies, each with a different intervention effect.[12] The separate funnels for each subgroup are symmetrical. Unfortunately, in practice, important sources of heterogeneity are often unknown.

Differences in methodological quality may also cause heterogeneity and lead to funnel plot asymmetry. Smaller studies tend to be conducted and analysed with less methodological rigour than larger studies,[13] and trials of lower quality also tend to show larger intervention effects.[14 15]

Reporting bias

Reporting biases arise when the dissemination of research findings is influenced by the nature and direction of results. Statistically significant "positive" results are more likely to be published, published rapidly, published in English, published more than once, published in high impact

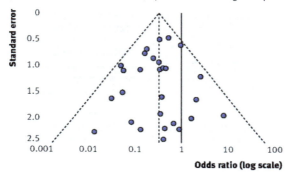

Fig 1 Example of symmetrical funnel plot. The outer dashed lines indicate the triangular region within which 95% of studies are expected to lie in the absence of both biases and heterogeneity (fixed effect summary log odds ratio±1.96×standard error of summary log odds ratio). The solid vertical line corresponds to no intervention effect

journals, and cited by others.[16 17 18 19] Data that would lead to negative results may be filtered, manipulated, or presented in such a way that they become positive.[14 20]

Reporting biases can have three types of consequence for a meta-analysis:

- A systematic review may fail to locate an eligible study because all information about it is suppressed or hard to find (publication bias)

- A located study may not provide usable data for the outcome of interest because the study authors did not consider the result sufficiently interesting (selective outcome reporting)

- A located study may provide biased results for some outcome—for example, by presenting the result with the smallest P value or largest effect estimate after trying several analysis methods (selective analysis reporting).

These biases may cause funnel plot asymmetry if statistically significant results suggesting a beneficial effect are more likely to be published than non-significant results. Such asymmetry may be exaggerated if there is a further tendency for smaller studies to be more prone to selective suppression of results than larger studies. This is often assumed to be the case for randomised trials. For instance, it is probably more difficult to make a large study disappear without trace, while a small study can easily be lost in a file drawer.[21] The same may apply to specific outcomes—for example, it is difficult not to report on mortality or myocardial infarction if these are outcomes of a large study.

Smaller studies have more sampling error in their effect estimates. Thus even though the risk of a false positive significant finding is the same, multiple analyses are more likely to yield a large effect estimate that may seem worth publishing. However, biases may not act this way in real life; funnel plots could be symmetrical even in the presence of publication bias or selective outcome reporting[19 22]— for example, if the published findings point to effects in different directions but unreported results indicate neither direction. Alternatively, bias may have affected few studies and therefore not cause glaring asymmetry.

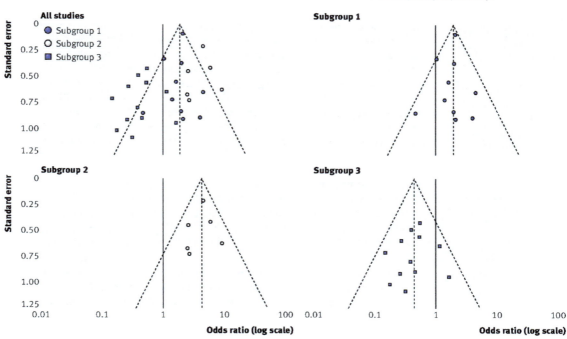

Fig 2 Illustration of funnel plot asymmetry due to heterogeneity, in the form of three distinct subgroups of studies. Funnel plot including all studies (top left) shows clear asymmetry (P<0.001 from Egger test for funnel plot asymmetry). P values for each subgroup are all >0.49.

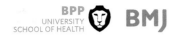

BOX 1 POSSIBLE SOURCES OF ASYMMETRY IN FUNNEL PLOTS
(ADAPTED FROM EGGER ET AL[1])

Reporting biases
- Publication bias:
  Delayed publication (also known as time lag or pipeline) bias
  Location biases (eg, language bias, citation bias, multiple publication bias)
- Selective outcome reporting
- Selective analysis reporting

Poor methodological quality leading to spuriously inflated effects in smaller studies
- Poor methodological design
- Inadequate analysis
- Fraud

True heterogeneity
- Size of effect differs according to study size (eg, because of differences in the intensity of interventions or in underlying risk between studies of different sizes)

Artefactual
- In some circumstances, sampling variation can lead to an association between the intervention effect and its standard error

Chance
- Asymmetry may occur by chance, which motivates the use of asymmetry tests

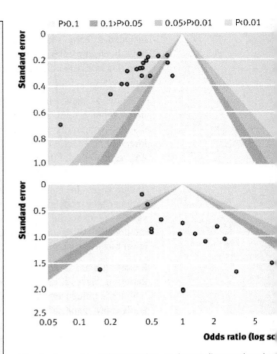

Fig 3 Contour enhanced funnel plots. In the top diagram there is a suggestion of missing studies in the middle and right of the plot, broadly in the white area of non-significance, making publication plausible. In the bottom diagram there is a suggestion of missing studies on the bottom left hand side of the plot. Since most of th[is] area contains regions of high significance, publication bias is unlik[ely] to be the underlying cause of asymmetry

Chance

The role of chance is critical for interpretation of funnel plots because most meta-analyses of randomised trials in healthcare contain few studies.[2] Investigations of relations across studies in a meta-analysis are seriously prone to false positive findings when there is a small number of studies and heterogeneity across studies,[23] and this may affect funnel plot symmetry.

Interpreting funnel plot asymmetry

Authors of systematic reviews should distinguish between possible reasons for funnel plot asymmetry (box 1). Knowledge of the intervention, and the circumstances in which it was implemented in different studies, can help identify causes of asymmetry in funnel plots, which should also be interpreted in the context of susceptibility to biases of research in the field of interest. Potential conflicts of interest, whether outcomes and analyses have been standardised, and extent of trial registration may need to be considered. For example, studies of antidepressants generate substantial conflicts of interest because the drugs generate vast sales revenues. Furthermore, there are hundreds of outcome scales, analyses can be very flexible, and trial registration was uncommon until recently.[24] Conversely, in a prospective meta-analysis where all data are included and all analyses fully standardised and conducted according to a predetermined protocol, publication or reporting biases cannot exist. Reporting bias is therefore more likely to be a cause of an asymmetric plot in the first situation than in the second.

Terrin et al found that researchers were poor at identifying publication bias from funnel plots.[5] Including contour lines corresponding to perceived milestones of statistical significance (P=0.01, 0.05, 0.1, etc) may aid visual interpretation.[25] If studies seem to be missing in areas of non-significance (fig 3, top) then asymmetry may be due to reporting bias, although other explanations should still be considered. If the supposed missing studies are in area[s of] higher significance or in a direction likely to be conside[red] desirable to their authors (fig 3, bottom), asymmetry [is] probably due to factors other than reporting bias.

Statistical tests for funnel plot asymmetry

A test for funnel plot asymmetry (sometimes referred to a[s a] test for small study effects) examines whether the associa[tion] between estimated intervention effects and a measure [of] study size is greater than might be expected to occur [by] chance. These tests typically have low power, so even w[hen] a test does not provide evidence of asymmetry, bias can[not] be excluded. For outcomes measured on a continuous s[cale] a test based on a weighted linear regression of the ef[fect] estimates on their standard errors is straightforward.[1] W[hen] outcomes are dichotomous and intervention effects [are] expressed as odds ratios, this corresponds to an inve[rse] variance weighted linear regression of the log odds r[atio] on its standard error.[2] Unfortunately, there are statist[ical] problems because the standard error of the log odds r[atio] is mathematically linked to the size of the odds ratio, e[ven] in the absence of small study effects.[2 4] Many authors h[ave] therefore proposed alternative tests (see appendix on b[mj.] com).[4 26 27 28]

Because it is impossible to know the pre[cise] mechanism(s) leading to funnel plot asymmetry, simula[ted] studies (in which tests are evaluated on large number[s of] computer generated datasets) are required to evaluate [their] characteristics. Most have examined a range of assumpti[ons] about the extent of reporting bias by selectively remov[ing] studies from simulated datasets.[26 27 28] After review[ing] the results of these studies, and based on theoret[ical] considerations, we formulated recommendations on test[s] for funnel plot asymmetry (box 2). The appendix descri[bes] the proposed tests, explains the reasons that some were [not] recommended, and discusses funnel plots for interven[tions]

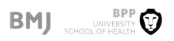

BOX 2 RECOMMENDATIONS ON TESTING FOR FUNNEL PLOT ASYMMETRY

All types of outcome

As a rule of thumb, tests for funnel plot asymmetry should not be used when there are fewer than 10 studies in the meta-analysis because test power is usually too low to distinguish chance from real asymmetry. (The lower the power of a test, the higher the proportion of "statistically significant" results in which there is in reality no association between study size and intervention effects). In some situations—for example, when there is substantial heterogeneity—the minimum number of studies may be substantially more than 10

Test results should be interpreted in the context of visual inspection of funnel plots— for example, are there studies with markedly different intervention effect estimates or studies that are highly influential in the asymmetry test? Even if an asymmetry test is statistically significant, publication bias can probably be excluded if small studies tend to lead to lower estimates of benefit than larger studies or if there are no studies with significant results

When there is evidence of funnel plot asymmetry, publication bias is only one possible explanation (see box 1)

As far as possible, testing strategy should be specified in advance: choice of test may depend on the degree of heterogeneity observed. Applying and reporting many tests is discouraged: if more than one test is used, all test results should be reported

Tests for funnel plot asymmetry should not be used if the standard errors of the intervention effect estimates are all similar (the studies are of similar sizes)

Continuous outcomes with intervention effects measured as mean differences

The test proposed by Egger et al may be used to test for funnel plot asymmetry.[1] There is no reason to prefer more recently proposed tests, although their relative advantages and disadvantages have not been formally examined. General considerations suggest that the power will be greater than for dichotomous outcomes but that use of the test with substantially fewer than 10 studies would be unwise

Dichotomous outcomes with intervention effects measured as odds ratios

The tests proposed by Harbord et al[26] and Peters et al[27] avoid the mathematical association between the log odds ratio and its standard error when there is a substantial intervention effect while retaining power compared with alternative tests. However, false positive results may still occur if there is substantial between study heterogeneity

If there is substantial between study heterogeneity (the estimated heterogeneity variance of log odds ratios, τ^2, is >0.1) only the arcsine test including random effects, proposed by Rücker et al, has been shown to work reasonably well.[28] However, it is slightly conservative in the absence of heterogeneity and its interpretation is less familiar than for other tests because it is based on an arcsine transformation.

When τ^2 is <0.1, one of the tests proposed by Harbord et al,[26] Peters et al,[27] or Rücker et al[28] can be used. Test performance generally deteriorates as τ^2 increases.

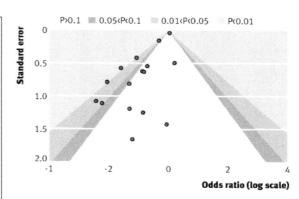

Fig 4 Contour enhanced funnel plot for trials of the effect of intravenous magnesium on mortality after myocardial infarction

effects measured as risk ratios, risk differences, and standardised mean differences. Our recommendations imply that tests for funnel plot asymmetry should be used in only a minority of meta-analyses.[29]

Funnel plots and meta-analysis models

Fixed and random effects models

Funnel plots can help guide choice of meta-analysis method. Random effects meta-analyses weight studies relatively more equally than fixed effect analyses by incorporating the between study variance into the denominator of each weight. If effect estimates are related to standard errors (funnel plot asymmetry), the random effects estimate will be pulled more towards findings from smaller studies than the fixed effect estimate will be. Random effects models can thus have undesirable consequences and are not always conservative.[30]

The trials of intravenous magnesium after myocardial infarction provide an extreme example of the differences between fixed and random effects analyses that can arise in the presence of funnel plot asymmetry.[31] Beneficial effects on mortality, found in a meta-analysis of small studies,[32] were subsequently contradicted when the very large ISIS-4 study found no evidence of benefit.[33] A contour enhanced funnel plot (fig 4) gives a clear visual impression of asymmetry, which is confirmed by small P values from the Harbord and Peters tests (P<0.001 and P=0.002 respectively).

Figure 5 shows that in a fixed effect analysis ISIS-4 receives 90% of the weight, and there is no evidence of a beneficial effect. However, there is clear evidence of between study heterogeneity (P<0.001, I^2=68%), and in a random effects analysis the small studies dominate so that intervention appears beneficial. To interpret the accumulated evidence, it is necessary to make a judgment about the validity or relevance of the combined evidence from the smaller studies compared with that from ISIS-4. The contour enhanced funnel plot suggests that publication bias does not completely explain the asymmetry, since many of the beneficial effects reported from smaller studies were not significant. Plausible explanations for these results are that methodological flaws in the smaller studies, or changes in the standard of care (widespread adoption of treatments such as aspirin, heparin, and thrombolysis), led to apparent beneficial effects of magnesium. This belief was reinforced by the subsequent publication of the MAGIC trial, in which magnesium added to these treatments which also found no evidence of benefit on mortality (odds ratio 1.0, 95% confidence interval 0.8 to 1.1).[34]

We recommend that when review authors are concerned about funnel plot asymmetry in a meta-analysis with evidence of between study heterogeneity, they should compare the fixed and random effects estimates of the intervention effect. If the random effects estimate is more beneficial, authors should consider whether it is plausible that the intervention is more effective in smaller studies. Formal investigations of heterogeneity of effects may reveal explanations for funnel plot asymmetry, in which case presentation of results should focus on these. If larger studies tend to be methodologically superior to smaller studies, or were conducted in circumstances more typical of the use of the intervention in practice, it may be appropriate to include only larger studies in the meta-analysis.

Extrapolation of a funnel plot regression line

An assumed relation between susceptibility to bias and study size can be exploited by extrapolating within a funnel plot. When funnel plot asymmetry is due to bias rather than substantive heterogeneity, it is usually assumed that results from larger studies are more believable than those from smaller studies because they are less susceptible to methodological flaws or reporting biases. Extrapolating a regression line on a funnel plot to minimum bias (maximum sample size) produces a meta-analytical estimate that can be regarded as corrected for such biases.[35][36][37] However, because it is difficult to distinguish between asymmetry due to bias and asymmetry due to heterogeneity or chance, the broad applicability of such approaches is uncertain. Further approaches to adjusting for publication bias are described and discussed in the appendix.

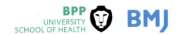

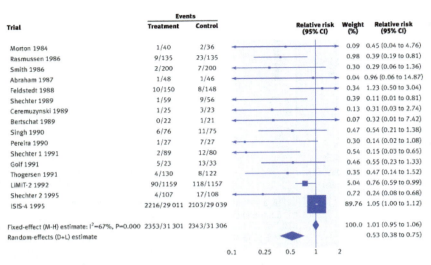

Trial	Events		Relative risk (95% CI)	Weight (%)	Relative risk (95% CI)
	Treatment	Control			
Morton 1984	1/40	2/36		0.09	0.45 (0.04 to 4.76)
Rasmussen 1986	9/135	23/135		0.98	0.39 (0.19 to 0.81)
Smith 1986	2/200	7/200		0.30	0.29 (0.06 to 1.36)
Abraham 1987	1/48	1/46		0.04	0.96 (0.06 to 14.87)
Feldstedt 1988	10/150	8/148		0.34	1.23 (0.50 to 3.04)
Shechter 1989	1/59	9/56		0.39	0.11 (0.01 to 0.81)
Ceremuzynski 1989	1/25	3/23		0.13	0.31 (0.03 to 2.74)
Bertschat 1989	0/22	1/21		0.07	0.32 (0.01 to 7.42)
Singh 1990	6/76	11/75		0.47	0.54 (0.21 to 1.38)
Pereira 1990	1/27	7/27		0.30	0.14 (0.02 to 1.08)
Shechter 1 1991	2/89	12/80		0.54	0.15 (0.03 to 0.65)
Golf 1991	5/23	13/33		0.46	0.55 (0.23 to 1.33)
Thogersen 1991	4/130	8/122		0.35	0.47 (0.14 to 1.52)
LIMIT-2 1992	90/1159	118/1157		5.04	0.76 (0.59 to 0.99)
Shechter 2 1995	4/107	17/108		0.72	0.24 (0.08 to 0.68)
ISIS-4 1995	2216/29 011	2103/29 039		89.76	1.05 (1.00 to 1.12)
Fixed-effect (M-H) estimate: I²=67%, P=0.000	2353/31 301	2343/31 306		100.0	1.01 (0.95 to 1.06)
Random-effects (D+L) estimate					0.53 (0.38 to 0.75)

Fig 5 Comparison of fixed and random effects meta-analytical estimates of the effect of intravenous magnesium on mortality after myocardial infarction

Discussion

Reporting biases are one of a number of possible explanations for the associations between study size and effect size that are displayed in asymmetric funnel plots. Examining and testing for funnel plot asymmetry, when appropriate, is an important means of addressing bias in meta-analyses, but the multiple causes of asymmetry and limited power of asymmetry tests mean that other ways to address reporting biases are also of importance. Searches of online trial registries can identify unpublished trials, although they do not currently guarantee access to trial protocols and results. When there are no registered but unpublished trials, and the outcome of interest is reported by all trials, restricting meta-analyses to registered trials should preclude publication bias. Recent comparisons of results of published trials with those submitted for regulatory approval have also provided clear evidence of reporting bias.[38] [39] Methods for dealing with selective reporting of outcomes have been described elsewhere.[40]

Our recommendations apply to meta-analyses of randomised trials, and their applicability in other contexts such as meta-analyses of epidemiological or diagnostic test studies is unclear.[41] The performance of tests for funnel plot asymmetry in these contexts is likely to differ from that in meta-analyses of randomised trials. Further factors, such as confounding and precision of measurements, may cause a relation between study size and effect estimates in observational studies. For example, large studies based on routinely collected data might not fully control confounding compared with smaller, purpose designed studies that collected a wide range of potential confounding variables. Alternatively, larger studies might use self reported exposure levels, which are more error prone, while smaller studies used precise measuring instruments. However, simulation studies have usually not considered such situations. An exception is for diagnostic studies, where large imbalances in group sizes and substantial odds ratios lead to poor performance of some tests: that proposed by Deeks et al was designed for use in this context.[4]

Contributors: All authors contributed to the drafting and editing of the manuscript. DA, JC, JD, RMH, JPTH, JPAI, DRJ, DM, JP, GR, JACS, AJS and JT contributed to the chapter in the *Cochrane Handbook for Systematic Reviews of Interventions* on which our recommendations on testing for funnel plot asymmetry are based. JACS will act as guarantor.

Funding: Funded in part by the Cochrane Collaboration Bias Methods Group, which receives infrastructure funding as part of a commitment by the Canadian Institutes of Health Research (CIHR) and the Canadian Agency for Drugs and Technologies in Health (CADTH) to fund Canadian based Cochrane entities. This supports dissemination activities, web hosting, travel, training, workshops and a full time coordinator position. JPTH was funded by MRC Grant U.1052.00.011. DGA is supported by Cancer Research UK. GR was supported by a grant from Deutsche Forschungsgemeinschaft (FOR 534 Schw 821/2-).

Competing interests. JC, JJD, SD, RMH, JPAI, DRJ, PM, JP, GR, GS, JACS and AJS are all authors on papers proposing tests for funnel plot asymmetry, but have no commercial interests in the use of these tests. All authors have completed the ICJME unified disclosure form at www.icmje.org/coi_disclosure.pdf (available on request from the corresponding author) and declare that they have no financial or non-financial interests that may be relevant to the submitted work.

Provenance and peer review: Not commissioned; externally peer reviewed.

1 Egger M, Davey Smith G, Schneider M, Minder C. Bias in meta-analysis detected by a simple, graphical test. *BMJ* 1997;315:629-34.
2 Sterne JAC, Gavaghan D, Egger M. Publication and related bias in meta-analysis: power of statistical tests and prevalence in the literature. *J Clin Epidemiol* 2000;53:1119-29.
3 Lau J, Ioannidis JP, Terrin N, Schmid CH, Olkin I. The case of the misleading funnel plot. *BMJ* 2006;333:597-600.
4 Deeks JJ, Macaskill P, Irwig L. The performance of tests of publication bias and other sample size effects in systematic reviews of diagnostic test accuracy was assessed. *J Clin Epidemiol* 2005;58:882-93.
5 Terrin N, Schmid CH, Lau J. In an empirical evaluation of the funnel plot, researchers could not visually identify publication bias. *J Clin Epidemiol* 2005;58:894-901.
6 Ioannidis JP. Interpretation of tests of heterogeneity and bias in meta-analysis. *J Eval Clin Pract* 2008;14:951-7.
7 Sterne JAC, Egger M, Moher D. Addressing reporting biases. In: Higgins JPT, Green S, eds. *Cochrane handbook for systematic reviews of interventions* . Wiley, 2008.
8 Sterne JAC, Egger M. Funnel plots for detecting bias in meta-analysis: guidelines on choice of axis. *J Clin Epidemiol* 2001;54:1046-55.
9 Begg CB, Berlin JA. Publication bias: a problem in interpreting medical data. *J R Statist Soc A* 1988;151:419-63.
10 Davey Smith G, Egger M. Who benefits from medical interventions? Treating low risk patients can be a high risk strategy. *BMJ* 1994;308:72-4.
11 Stuck AE, Siu AL, Wieland GD, Adams J, Rubenstein LZ. Comprehensive geriatric assessment: a meta-analysis of controlled trials. *Lancet* 1993;342:1032-6.
12 Peters JL, Sutton AJ, Jones DR, Abrams KR, Rushton L, Moreno SG. Assessing publication bias in meta-analyses in the presence of between-study heterogeneity. *J R Statist Soc A* 2010;173:575-91.
13 Egger M, Jüni P, Bartlett C, Holenstein F, Sterne J. How important are comprehensive literature searches and the assessment of trial quality in systematic reviews? Empirical study. *Health Technol Assess* 2003;7:1-68.
14 Ioannidis JP. Why most discovered true associations are inflated. *Epidemiology* 2008;19:640-8.
15 Wood L, Egger M, Gluud LL, Schulz KF, Jüni P, Altman DG, et al. Empirical evidence of bias in treatment effect estimates in controlled trials with different interventions and outcomes: meta-epidemiological study. *BMJ* 2008;336:601-5.
16 Hopewell S, Clarke M, Stewart L, Tierney J. Time to publication for results of clinical trials. *Cochrane Database Syst Rev* 2007;2:MR000011.
17 Hopewell S, Loudon K, Clarke MJ, Oxman AD, Dickersin K. Publication bias in clinical trials due to statistical significance or direction of trial results. *Cochrane Database Syst Rev* 2009;1:MR000006.
18 Song F, Parekh S, Hooper L, Loke YK, Ryder J, Sutton J, et al. Dissemination and publication of research findings: an updated review of related biases. *Health Technol Assess* 2010;14:iii,ix-iii,193.
19 Dwan K, Altman DG, Arnaiz JA, Bloom J, Chan AW, Cronin E, et al. Systematic review of the empirical evidence of study publication bias and outcome reporting bias. *PLoS ONE* 2008;3:e3081.
20 Turner EH, Matthews AM, Linardatos E, Tell RA, Rosenthal R. Selective publication of antidepressant trials and its influence on apparent efficacy. *N Engl J Med* 2008;358:252-60.
21 Rosenthal R. The "file drawer" problem and tolerance for null results. *Psychol Bull* 1979;86:638-41.
22 Chan AW, Hrobjartsson A, Haahr MT, Gotzsche PC, Altman DG. Empirical evidence for selective reporting of outcomes in randomized trials: comparison of protocols to published articles. *JAMA* 2004;291:2457-65.
23 Higgins JP, Thompson SG. Controlling the risk of spurious findings from meta-regression. *Stat Med* 2004;23:1663-82.
24 Ioannidis JP. Effectiveness of antidepressants: an evidence myth constructed from a thousand randomized trials? *Philos Ethics Humanit Med* 2008;3:14.
25 Peters J, Sutton AJ, Jones DR, Abrams KR, Rushton L. Contour-enhanced meta-analysis funnel plots help distinguish publication bias from other causes of asymmetry. *J Clin Epidemiol* 2008;61:991-6.

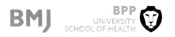

26 Harbord RM, Egger M, Sterne JA. A modified test for small-study effects in meta-analyses of controlled trials with binary endpoints. *Stat Med* 2006;25:3443-57.

27 Peters JL, Sutton AJ, Jones DR, Abrams KR, Rushton L. Comparison of two methods to detect publication bias in meta-analysis. *JAMA* 2006;295:676-80.

28 Rücker G, Schwarzer G, Carpenter J. Arcsine test for publication bias in meta-analyses with binary outcomes. *Stat Med* 2008;27:746-63.

29 Ioannidis JP, Trikalinos TA. The appropriateness of asymmetry tests for publication bias in meta-analyses: a large survey. *CMAJ* 2007;176:1091-6.

30 Poole C, Greenland S. Random-effects meta-analyses are not always conservative. *Am J Epidemiol* 1999;150:469-75.

31 Egger M, Davey Smith G. Misleading meta-analysis. Lessons from an "effective, safe, simple" intervention that wasn't. *BMJ* 1995;310:752-4.

32 Teo KK, Yusuf S, Collins R, Held PH, Peto R. Effects of intravenous magnesium in suspected acute myocardial infarction: overview of randomised trials. *BMJ* 1991;303:1499-503.

33 ISIS-4 (Fourth International Study of Infarct Survival) Collaborative Group. ISIS-4: a randomised factorial trial assessing early oral captopril, oral mononitrate, and intravenous magnesium sulphate in 58,050 patients with suspected acute myocardial infarction. *Lancet* 1995;345:669-85.

34 Early administration of intravenous magnesium to high-risk patients with acute myocardial infarction in the Magnesium in Coronaries (MAGIC) Trial: a randomised controlled trial. *Lancet* 2002;360:1189-96.

35 Shang A, Huwiler-Muntener K, Nartey L, Jüni P, Dörig S, Stene JA, et al. Are the clinical effects of homoeopathy placebo effects? Comparative study of placebo-controlled trials of homoeopathy and allopathy. *Lancet* 2005;366:726-32.

36 Moreno SG, Sutton AJ, Ades AE, Stanley TD, Abrams KR, Peters JL, et al. Assessment of regression-based methods to adjust for publication bias through a comprehensive simulation study. *BMC Med Res Methodol* 2009;9:2.

37 Rucker G, Schwarzer G, Carpenter JR, Binder H, Schumacher M. Treatment-effect estimates adjusted for small-study effects via a limit meta-analysis. *Biostatistics* 2011;12:122-42.

38 Moreno SG, Sutton AJ, Turner EH, Abrams KR, Cooper NJ, Palmer TM, et al. Novel methods to deal with publication biases: secondary analysis of antidepressant trials in the FDA trial registry database and related journal publications. *BMJ* 2009;339:b2981.

39 Eyding D, Lelgemann M, Grouven U, Härter M, Kromp M, Kaiser T, et al. Reboxetine for acute treatment of major depression: systematic review and meta-analysis of published and unpublished placebo and selective serotonin reuptake inhibitor controlled trials. *BMJ* 2010;341:c4737.

40 Kirkham JJ, Dwan KM, Altman DG, Gamble C, Dodd S, Smyth R, et al. The impact of outcome reporting bias in randomised controlled trials on a cohort of systematic reviews. *BMJ* 2010;340:c365.

41 Egger M, Schneider M, Davey Smith G. Spurious precision? Meta-analysis of observational studies. *BMJ* 1998;316:140-4.

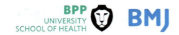

Brackets (parentheses) in formulas

Douglas G Altman, professor of statistics in medicine[1],
J Martin Bland, professor of health statistics[2]

[1]Centre for Statistics in Medicine, University of Oxford, Oxford OX2 6UD

[2]Department of Health Sciences, University of York, York YO10 5DD

Correspondence to: DG Altman doug. altman@csm.ox.ac.uk

Cite this as: *BMJ* 2011;343:d570

DOI: 10.1136/bmj.d570

http://www.bmj.com/content/343/bmj.d570

Each year, new health sciences postgraduate students in York are given a simple maths test. Each year the majority of them fail to calculate $20 - 3 \times 5$ correctly. According to the conventional rules of arithmetic, division and multiplication are done before addition and subtraction, so $20 - 3 \times 5 = 20 - 15 = 5$. Many students work from left to right and calculate $20 - 3 \times 5$ as $17 \times 5 = 85$. If that was what was actually meant, we would need to use brackets: $(20 - 3) \times 5 = 17 \times 5 = 85$. Brackets tell us that the enclosed part must be evaluated first. That convention is part of various mnemonic acronyms which indicate the order of operations, such as BODMAS (Brackets, Of (that is, power of), Divide, Multiply, Add, Subtract) and PEMDAS (Parentheses, Exponentiation, Multiplication, Division, Addition, Subtraction).[1]

Schoolchildren learn the basic rules about how to construct and interpret mathematical formulas.[1] The conventions exist to ensure that there is absolutely no ambiguity, as mathematics (unlike prose) has no redundancy, so any mistake may have serious consequences. Our experience is that mistakes are quite common when formulas are presented in medical journal articles. A particular concern is that brackets are often omitted or misused. The following examples are typical and we mean nothing personal by choosing them.

Example 1

In a discussion of methods for analysing diagnostic test accuracy, Collinson[2] wrote:

Sensitivity = TP/TP + FN

where TP = true positive and FN = false negative. The formula should, of course, be:

Sensitivity = TP/(TP + FN).

Example 2

For a non-statistical example, Leyland[3] wrote that the total optical power of the cornea is:

$P = P_1 + P_2 - t/n_2 (P_1 P_2)$

where $P_1 = n_2 - n_1/r_1$ and $P_2 = n_3 - n_2/r_2$. Here n_1, n_2, and n_3 are refractive indices, r_1, r_2, and t are distances in metres, and P, P_1, and P_2, are powers in dioptres. But he should have written $P_1 = (n_2 - n_1)/r_1$ and $P_2 = (n_3 - n_2)/r2$. $P_1 = n_2 - n_1/r_1$ is clearly wrong dimensionally, as P_1 is dioptres, 1/metre, n_2 and n_1 are ratios and so pure numbers, and r_1 is in metres. Also, it is not clear whether $t/n_2 (P_1 P_2)$ means $(t/n_2) P_1 P_2$, which it does, or $t/(n_2 P_1 P_2)$.

Do such errors matter? Certainly. In our experience the calculations are usually correct in the paper, but anyone using the published formula would go wrong. Sometimes, however, the incorrect formula was used, as in the following case.

Example 3

In their otherwise exemplary evaluation of the chronic ankle instability scale, Eechaute et al[4] made a mistake in their formula for the minimal detectable change (MDC) or repeatability coefficient,[5] writing: MDC = $2.04 \times (2 \times SE$ Here SEM is the standard error of a measurement or wi subject standard deviation.[5] This formula uses 2.04 wh 2 or 1.96 is more usual,[6] but, much more seriously, SEM should not be included within the square root, as brackets indicate. This might be dismissed as a sim typographical error, but the authors actually used incorrect formula. Their value of SEM was 2.7 points, they calculated the minimal detectable change as 2.0 $(2 \times 2.7) = 4.7$. They should have calculated $2.04 \times (2$ $2.7 = 7.8$. Their erroneous formula makes the scale app considerably more reliable than it actually is.[6] The form is also wrong in terms of dimensions, because the minim clinical difference should be in the same units as measurement, not in square root units.

Some mistakes in formulas may be present in submitted manuscript, but others might be introduced the publication process. For example, problems sometir arise when a displayed formula is converted to an "in-te formula as part of the editing, and the implications are realised or not noticed by either editing staff or auth Often it is necessary to insert brackets when reformattin formula. So the simple formula:

$$\frac{p}{1 - p}$$

should be changed to $p/(1 - p)$ if moved to the text.

Formulas in published articles may be used by othe so mistakes may lead to substantive errors in resear It is essential that authors and editors check all formu carefully.

Acknowledgements: We are very grateful to Phil McShane for point out a mistake in an earlier version of this statistics note.

Contributors: DGA and JMB jointly wrote and agreed the text.

Competing interests: All authors have completed the Unified Competing Interest form at www.icmje.org/coi_disclosure.pdf (available on request from the corresponding author) and declare: no support from any organisation for the submitted; no financial relationships with any organisations that might have an interest in the submitted work in the previous 3 years; no other relationships activities that could appear to have influenced the submitted work

1 Wikipedia. Order of operations. [cited 2010 Nov 23]. http://en.wikipedia.org/wiki/Order_of_operations
2 Collinson P. Of bombers, radiologists, and cardiologists: time to RO *Heart* 1998;80:215-7.
3 Leyland M. Validation of Orbscan II posterior corneal curvature measurement for intraocular lens power calculation. *Eye* 2004;18:357-60.
4 Eechaute C, Vaes P, Duquet W. The chronic ankle instability scale: Clinimetric properties of a multidimensional, patient-assessed instrument. *Phys Ther Sport* 2008;9:57-66.
5 Bland JM, Altman DG. Statistics Notes. Measurement error. *BMJ* 1996;312:744.
6 Bland JM. Minimal detectable change. *Phys Ther Sport* 2009;10:39.

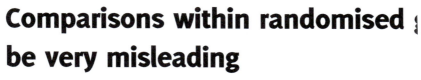

Comparisons within randomised be very misleading

J Martin Bland, professor of health statistics[1],
Douglas G Altman, professor of statistics in medicine[2]

partment of Health Sciences,
versity of York, York YO10 5DD

ntre for Statistics in Medicine,
versity of Oxford, Oxford OX2

espondence to: Professor M
d martin.bland@york.ac.uk

this as: BMJ 2011;342:d561

10.1136/bmj.d561

://www.bmj.com/content/342/
.d561

When we randomise trial participants into two or more intervention groups, we do this to remove bias; the groups will, on average, be comparable in every respect except the treatment which they receive. Provided the trial is well conducted, without other sources of bias, any difference in the outcome of the groups can then reasonably be attributed to the different interventions received. In a previous note we discussed the analysis of those trials in which the primary outcome measure is also measured at baseline. We discussed several valid analyses, observing that "analysis of covariance" (a regression method) is the method of choice.[1]

Rather than comparing the randomised groups directly, however, researchers sometimes look at the change in the measurement between baseline and the end of the trial; they test whether there was a significant change from baseline, separately in each randomised group. They may then report that this difference is significant in one group but not in the other, and conclude that this is evidence that the groups, and hence the treatments, are different.

One such example was a recent trial in which participants were randomised to receive either an "anti-ageing" cream or the vehicle as a placebo.[2] A wrinkle score was recorded at baseline and after six months. The authors gave the results of significance tests comparing the score with baseline for each group separately, reporting the active treatment group to have a significant difference (P=0.013) and the vehicle group not (P=0.11). Their interpretation was that the cosmetic cream resulted in significant clinical improvement in facial wrinkles. But we cannot validly draw this conclusion, because the lack of a significant difference in the vehicle group does not provide good evidence that the anti-ageing product is superior.[3]

The essential feature of a randomised trial is the comparison *between* groups. Within group analyses do not address a meaningful question: the question is not whether there is a change from baseline, but whether any change is greater in one group than the other. It is not possible to draw valid inferences by comparing P values. In particular, there is an inflated risk of a false positive result, which we shall illustrate with a simulation.

The table shows simulated data for a randomised trial with two groups of 30 participants. Data were drawn from the same population, so there is no systematic difference between the two groups. The true baseline measurements had a mean of 10.0 with standard deviation (SD) 2.0, and the outcome measurement was equal to the baseline plus an increase of 0.5 and a random element with SD 1.0. The difference between mean outcomes is 0.22 (95% confidence interval –0.75 to 0.34, P=0.5), adjusting for the baseline by analysis of covariance.[1] The difference is not statistically significant, which is not surprising because we know that the null hypothesis of no difference in the population is true. If we compare baseline with outcome for each group using a paired t test, however, for group A the difference is statistically significant, P=0.03, for group B it is not significant, P = 0.2. These results are quite similar to those of the anti-ageing cream trial.[2]

We would not wish to draw any conclusions from one simulation. In 1000 runs, the difference between groups had P<0.05 in the analysis of covariance 47 times, or for 4.7% of samples, very close to the 5% we expect. Of the 2000 comparisons between baseline and outcome, 1500 (75%) had P<0.05. In this simulation, where there is no difference whatsoever between the two "treatments," the probability of a significant difference in one group but not the other was 38%, not 5%. Hence a significant difference in one group but not the other is not good evidence of a significant difference between the groups. Even when there is a clear benefit of one treatment over the other, separate P values are not the way to analyse such studies.[4]

How many pairs of tests will have one significant and one non-significant difference depends on the size of the change from baseline to final measurement. If the population difference from baseline is very large, nearly

le Simulated data from a randomised trial comparing two groups of 30 patients, with a true ange from baseline but no difference between groups (sorted by baseline values within each up)

	Group A				Group B		
	Baseline	6 months	Change		Baseline	6 months	Change
1	6.4	7.1	0.7	1	6.8	7.9	1.1
2	6.6	5.6	-1.0	2	7.2	7.5	0.3
3	7.3	8.3	1.0	3	7.2	6.9	-0.3
4	7.7	9.1	1.4	4	7.4	6.9	-0.5
5	7.7	9.5	1.8	5	7.5	8.3	0.8
6	7.9	9.6	1.7	6	7.5	9.4	1.9
7	8.0	8.5	0.5	7	8.3	9.0	0.7
8	8.0	8.5	0.5	8	8.4	8.8	0.4
9	8.1	9.1	1.0	9	8.7	8.0	-0.7
10	9.2	9.6	0.4	10	9.0	7.2	-1.8
11	9.3	8.7	-0.6	11	9.2	7.1	-2.1
12	9.6	10.7	1.1	12	9.6	10.6	1.0
13	9.7	9.0	-0.7	13	9.9	11.0	1.1
14	9.8	9.0	-0.8	14	10.1	11.5	1.4
15	9.8	8.0	-1.8	15	10.2	10.4	0.2
16	10.2	11.1	0.9	16	10.3	11.0	0.7
17	10.3	11.5	1.2	17	10.4	9.9	-0.5
18	10.6	9.1	-1.5	18	10.5	11.3	0.8
19	10.6	12.0	1.4	19	10.7	9.9	-0.8
20	10.7	13.2	2.5	20	10.8	10.7	-0.1
21	10.9	9.7	-1.2	21	10.8	11.8	1.0
22	11.1	12.2	1.1	22	11.1	10.0	-1.1
23	11.2	10.8	-0.4	23	11.1	13.2	2.1
24	11.8	11.9	0.1	24	11.4	11.8	0.4
25	12.3	12.2	-0.1	25	11.6	12.1	0.5
26	12.4	12.6	0.2	26	11.7	11.5	-0.2
27	13.1	15.0	1.9	27	12.0	12.7	0.7
28	13.2	13.8	0.6	28	12.3	13.7	1.4
29	13.3	14.1	0.8	29	13.7	12.6	-1.1
30	13.7	14.2	0.5	30	13.9	13.7	-0.2
ean	10.02	10.46	0.44	Mean	9.98	10.21	0.24
)	2.06	2.29	1.06	SD	1.90	2.09	1.02

all the within group tests will be significant, and if the population difference is small, nearly all tests will be not significant, so there will be few samples with only one significant difference. If the difference is such that half the samples would show a significant change from baseline, as it would be in our simulation if the underlying difference were 0.37 rather than 0.5, we would expect 50% of samples to have just one significant difference.

The anti-ageing trial is not the only one where we have seen this misleading approach applied to randomised trial data.[3] We even found it once in the *BMJ*[5]

Contributors: JMB and DGA jointly wrote and agreed the text, JMB did the statistical analysis.

Competing interests: All authors have completed the Unified Competing Interest form at www.icmje.org/coi_disclosure.pdf (available on request from the corresponding author) and declare: no support from any organisation for the submitted work; no financial relationships with any organisations that might have an interest in the submitted work in the previous 3 years; no other relationships or activities that could appear to have influenced the submitted work.

1   Vickers AJ, Altman DG. Analysing controlled trials with baseline and follow-up measurements. *BMJ* 2001;323:1123-4.
2   Watson REB, Ogden S, Cotterell LF, Bowden JJ, Bastrilles JY, Long SP, et al. A cosmetic 'anti-ageing' product improves photoaged skin: a double-blind, randomized controlled trial. *Br J Dermatol* 2009;161:419-26.
3   Bland JM. Evidence for an 'anti-ageing' product may not be so clear as it appears. *Br J Dermatol* 2009;161:1207-8.
4   Altman DG, Bland JM. Interaction revisited: the difference between two estimates. *BMJ* 2003;326:219.
5   Bland JM, Altman DG. Informed consent. *BMJ* 1993;306:928.

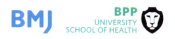

Uncertainties in baseline risk estimates and confidence in treatment effects

Frederick A Spencer, professor of medicine[1], Alfonso Iorio, associate professor of clinical epidemiology and biostatistics[1][2], John You, assistant professor of medicine[1][2], M Hassad Murad, associate professor of medicine[3], Holger J Schünemann, professor and chair of clinical epidemiology and biostatistics[1][2], Per O Vandvik, associate professor of medicine[4][5], Mark A Crowther, professor of medicine and molecular medicine[1][6], Kevin Pottie, associate professor of family medicine and epidemiology and community medicine[7], Eddy S Lang, senior researcher[8], Joerg J Meerpohl, deputy director of German Cochrane Centre[9], Yngve Falck-Ytter, assistant professor of medicine[10], Pablo Alonso-Coello, senior researcher[11], Gordon H Guyatt, professor of medicine and clinical epidemiology and biostatistics[2]

artment of Medicine,
aster University, Hamilton ON
1A6, Canada

artment of Clinical
emiology and Biostatistics,
aster University, Hamilton

sion of Preventive Medicine,
o Clinic, Rochester, Minnesota,

artment of Medicine, Inlandet
ital Trust, Gjøvik, Norway

wegian Knowledge Centre for
h Services, Oslo, Norway

artment of Molecular
icine, McMaster University,
ilton

artments of Family Medicine
Epidemiology and Community
icine, University of Ottawa,
wa, Canada

sion of Emergency Medicine,
ersity of Calgary, Calgary,
ada

nan Cochrane Center, Institute
edical Biometry and Medical
rmatics, University Medical
er, Freiburg, Germany

partment of Medicine, Case
ern Reserve University,
eland, USA

roamerican Cochrane Centre,
RESP-IIB Sant Pau, Barcelona,
n

espondence to: F A Spencer
nce@mcmaster.ca

this as: BMJ 2012;345:e7401

10.1136/bmj.e7401

//www.bmj.com/content/345/
e7401

The GRADE system provides a framework for assessing confidence in estimates of the effect ("quality of evidence") of alternative management strategies on outcomes that are important to patients.[1][2][3][4][5][6] The GRADE system includes consideration of risk of bias, publication bias, imprecision, inconsistency, and indirectness and their impact on confidence in estimates of benefits and harms. The evaluation of each of these issues has, thus far, focused almost exclusively on their potential impact on estimates of relative effect. Because, in most instances, estimates of relative effect of a therapy are similar across different baseline risks, one can apply these relative estimates to the best estimates of overall baseline risk or, if available, estimates from subgroups that differ in baseline risk.

Using the GRADE approach, guideline panellists multiply the best estimate of relative effect by the best available estimate of baseline risk to obtain an estimate of absolute effect (see box). Limitations of the evidence with respect to risk of bias, publication bias, imprecision, inconsistency, or indirectness may reduce confidence in estimates of the relative risk reduction and affect the strength of guideline recommendations.

As with estimates of relative effect, the quality of evidence supporting estimates of baseline risk can vary. At present, GRADE—and all other systems that address confidence in estimates of treatment effect—fails to fully explore issues of confidence in estimates of baseline risk. Nor do these

ABSTRACT

The GRADE system provides a framework for evaluating how risk of bias, publication bias, imprecision, inconsistency, and indirectness may reduce confidence in estimates of relative effects of interventions on outcomes. However, GRADE and all other systems for rating confidence in effect estimates do not fully address uncertainty in baseline risk and its impact on confidence in absolute estimates of treatment effect. In this article the authors examine factors that may reduce confidence in estimates of baseline risk and thus estimates of absolute treatment benefit

systems incorporate the 95% confidence interval of a baseline risk estimate when deriving their absolute risk estimates. Thus, evaluating uncertainty in baseline risk, and its impact on confidence in absolute estimates of treatment effect, remains an important outstanding issue.

We suggest that the domains currently used in GRADE (risk of bias, publication bias, imprecision, inconsistency, and indirectness) can also help to understand issues of confidence in baseline risk estimates. In this article we use examples from the *Antithrombotic Therapy and Prevention of Thrombosis, 9th edition* (AT9) to examine how these issues may influence estimates of baseline risk and the subsequent impact on derived estimates of absolute effect.

Risk of bias

In addressing treatment effects, evidence from observational studies generally warrants lower confidence than evidence from randomised controlled trials. However, community based or population based observational studies can provide better estimates of the baseline risk associated with a given clinical condition than randomised controlled trials, which often enrol highly selected populations. This will be true, however, only if the relevant observational studies are at low risk of bias in ascertaining event rates.

In the AT9 guidelines addressing atrial fibrillation,[7] the panellists derived baseline risk estimates of non-fatal stroke for patients with atrial fibrillation from pooled event rates in the control arms of six randomised controlled trials conducted in the early 1990s.[8] The panellists acknowledged limitations in these estimates, including the fact that the trials enrolled less than 10% of patients screened.

SUMMARY BOX

- Uncertainty in baseline risk estimates and its impact on confidence in absolute estimates of treatment effect are not adequately evaluated in systems of judging confidence in estimates of treatment effect—including GRADE
- Risk of bias, publication bias, imprecision, inconsistency, and indirectness can affect confidence in estimates of baseline risk and subsequently confidence in derived estimates of absolute effect of diagnostic and treatment modalities
- GRADE's structure can be easily and effectively adapted to better understand issues regarding confidence in baseline risk. Concerns can be categorised into one or more of the same domains used by GRADE to evaluate evidence supporting a relative risk estimate

In addition, the authors noted that more recent data from a large administrative database including a broader spectrum of patients suggested lower rates of non-fatal thromboembolism in untreated patients (4.2 v 2.1 per 100 patient years).[9] These lower rates may be more reflective of event rates in the current era and would make an important difference in the estimated absolute risk reduction (that is, a more modest effect) associated with anticoagulation in this class of patients.

The panel chose, however, to rely on the trial data because of concern that the lower estimate of stroke derived from the large administrative database reflected under-ascertainment of stroke (that is, a high risk of bias).

Publication bias

Relative risk estimates for the impact of a therapeutic strategy in relation to a comparator on a target outcome are ideally drawn from a systematic review of relevant studies. These estimates are biased if the included studies are unrepresentative because of preferential publication of studies favouring a stronger or weaker effect.[10] [11] In GRADE, systematic review and guideline authors may rate down their confidence in effect estimates if they believe publication bias is likely.[12]

Publication bias may similarly affect estimates of baseline risk. Ideally, systematic reviews of large observational studies including a representative sample of the target population will inform estimates of baseline risk. However, observational studies reporting higher undesirable event rates may be less likely to be published than studies reporting lower event rates. This may be particularly true for surgical series, in which surgeons experiencing a higher rate of adverse events than their colleagues may be reluctant to display their less enviable record to the surgical world.

Imprecision

Examination of 95% confidence intervals for estimates of absolute effects provides the optimal approach to determine precision of the estimate.[13] For practice guidelines, rating down the confidence in absolute estimates of effect is warranted if clinical action would differ if the upper versus the lower boundary of the confidence interval represented the truth.

Imprecision in estimates of baseline risk will affect the derived absolute effect of a given therapy. The AT9 guidelines suggest venous thromboprophylaxis with low dose, low molecular weight heparin (LMWH) for women undergoing assisted reproduction who develop severe ovarian hyperstimulation syndrome.[14] The authors estimate that use of low dose LMWH will prevent 26 venous thromboembolic events (95% confidence interval 13 to 42) per 1000 patients treated. Their estimate comes from applying indirect evidence of the relative risk reduction associated with low dose LMWH from existing surgical literature (relative risk 0.36 (95% confidence interval 0.20 to 0.67)) to a baseline venous thromboembolic event rate of 4.1%. The quality of evidence for the resulting recommendation was rated down for indirectness (relative risk estimate derived from a general surgical population).

This baseline risk of 4.1% was, however, derived from a sample of just 49 patients with severe ovarian hyperstimulation syndrome from a cohort of 2748 cycles of assisted reproduction therapy.[15] The 95% confidence interval around the 4.1% point estimate is 1.1% to 13.7%. Therefore, depending on selection of baseline risk (and multiplying by the 95% confidence interval of the relative risk reduction),

use of low dose LMWH in such patients may result in few as four events prevented to as many as 110 eve prevented per 1000 treated. The lower estimate of events per 1000 treated would make any recommenda for thromboprophylaxis in this population far less attrac than the latter. Such imprecision is likely to arise in conditions.

Inconsistency

In GRADE, confidence in estimates of effect from a bod evidence may be rated down if the magnitude of treatm effect varies substantially across relevant studie Inconsistency may also undermine estimates of base risk. Guideline developers often derive baseline estimates by pooling event rates from observational stud using similar populations. Event rates among indivic studies may vary greatly from the pooled estimate, t decreasing confidence in this estimate.

In the chapter of the AT9 guidelines address prophylaxis for venous thromboembolism in surg patients, the authors suggest an average risk of 2 for venous thromboembolism in patients undergo craniotomy and suggest use of lower extremity exte compression devices as prophylaxis.[17] This risk estim was derived from a pooled estimate of event rates obser in eight studies providing event rates in neurosurg patients using external compression devices.[18] Based this estimate, and multiplying by a relative risk estim of 0.56, the authors calculated that use of LMWH inst of external compression devices would prevent nine n fatal symptomatic venous thromboembolic events per 1 patients treated. Using a similar approach, they calcula that LMWH will cause 11 more non-fatal intracranial blee Based on these estimates of absolute benefit and ha they provided a weak recommendation for mechan prophylaxis over LMWH for venous thromboembolism.

The venous thromboembolic event rates in the inclu studies varied from 0% to 10%. This inconsiste decreases our confidence in the baseline risk estima and consequently in the recommendation. If true ven thromboembolic event rates are closer to 10% despite of external compression devices, LMWH would prevent non-fatal venous thromboembolic events per 1000 trea Based on this estimate of absolute effect, it is less c which prophylactic strategy should be recommended.

Indirectness

Direct evidence in the GRADE framework includes stud that have enrolled the populations of interest, delive the intervention in the manner of interest, and measu the outcomes important to patients over the time fra of interest.[19] A guideline panel will have concerns ab indirectness when the population, intervention, or outc differs from those in which they are interested—what might otherwise call limitations of applicability.

The evidence supporting a baseline risk estimate can a be indirect. This occurs when baseline risk estimates derived from a population that differs significantly from population to whom the resulting guidelines are direct Given the lack of high quality evidence documen outcome event rates for specific disease states in commu settings, estimates of baseline risks for outcome eve are often derived from event rates in the control arms randomised controlled trials. In general, patients enrol in such trials are younger, have less comorbidity, and h better outcomes than patients encountered in clin practice. Therefore, application of relative risk estima

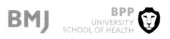

for a given intervention to a baseline risk rate derived from a randomised controlled trial may underestimate both the absolute benefits and harms associated with that intervention in the community setting.

Indirectness may also lead to overestimates of absolute effects. As discussed above, baseline risk estimates of non-fatal stroke for patients with atrial fibrillation in the AT9 guidelines were derived from the pooled event rates in the control arms of six randomised controlled trials comparing warfarin with aspirin in the early 1990s.[2] For CHADS2 (stroke risk) scores of 0, 1, 2, and 3-6, respectively, baseline event rates of 0.8%, 2.2%, 4.5%, and 9.6% per year were used to generate estimates of absolute benefit with warfarin. Rates of non-fatal thromboembolism in untreated patients were significantly lower in a more current and representative population than seen in the older trials (for CHADS2 scores of 0, 1, 2, 3, and 4-6, respectively, absolute event rates of 0.4%, 1.2%, 2.5%, 3.9%, and 6.3% were reported).[9]

Use of the estimates from the more current observational database would have resulted in a substantial decrease in the calculated absolute benefit of warfarin over one year. For example, using the baseline risk estimates from the older trials, warfarin use is predicted to prevent 30 non-fatal strokes per 1000 (95% confidence interval 23 to 35 strokes prevented) in patients with a CHADS2 score of 2. With the lower baseline risk estimates, however, the absolute benefit of warfarin decreases—resulting in prevention of only 16 (13 to 19) non-fatal thromboembolic events per 1000 treated. Similarly, absolute benefit for patients with a CHADS2 score of 1 would have declined from 15 (11 to 17) fewer events to eight (6 to 9) fewer events without a change in estimated harm due to bleeding. These revised absolute benefits would potentially alter recommendations—possibly changing the direction of the recommendation for warfarin in patients with a CHADS2 score of 1 and reducing the strength of the recommendation from strong to weak for warfarin over aspirin in patients with a CHADS2 score of 2.

Discussion

Adopted by over 60 groups worldwide, the GRADE approach represents an important innovation in interpreting evidence from systematic reviews, health technology assessments, and clinical practice guidelines. At present, the approach focuses on evaluating confidence in estimates in the relative effect of one treatment strategy over another, and then—in most cases—assuming that this confidence also applies to estimates of absolute effects. Estimates of baseline risks,

however, directly affect estimates of absolute risks and benefits of a treatment. We suggest that the confidence in estimates of baseline risks is subject to the same issues as evidence for relative effects of a treatment strategy.

To date guidelines have rarely considered issues of baseline risk. As our examples illustrate, GRADE's structure can be usefully adapted to better understand issues regarding confidence in baseline risk.

This discussion has only illustrated the problem. We are not yet ready to offer specific guidance on how to rate down confidence in estimates of baseline risk. As with other methodological problems previously encountered, a great deal of work studying specific examples needs to be done before we can offer concrete solutions. This article represents a first step in this process.

Contributors: FAS and GHG conceived the study and take responsibility for the integrity of the data and the accuracy of the data analysis. FAS is the guarantor. FAS, AI, and GHG designed the study. FAS, AI, JY, MHM, POV, and GHG analysed and interpreted the data. FAS, AI, MHM, and GHG drafted the manuscript. All authors critically revised the manuscript.

Funding: This study was not externally funded.

Competing interests: All authors have completed the ICMJE uniform disclosure form at www.icmje.org/coi_disclosure.pdf (available on request from the corresponding author) and declare: no support from any organisation for the submitted work; no financial relationships with any organisations that might have an interest in the submitted work in the previous three years; all authors are members of the GRADE working group and were contributors to *Antithrombotic Therapy and Prevention of Thrombosis, 9th edition*, but this manuscript is not submitted on behalf of either group.

Ethical approval: Not required.

Provenance: All authors were contributors to the *Antithrombotic Therapy and Prevention of Thrombosis, 9th edition*, which used the GRADE system to assess quality of evidence underlying subsequent recommendations. During the development of these guidelines, authors (in particular FAS, AI, POV, and GHG) struggled with issues of confidence in estimates of baseline risk and how to evaluate and categorise uncertainty in baseline risk estimates. Further discussion of these issues among panel members prompted the development of this manuscript.

1 Guyatt GH, Oxman AD, Schunemann HJ, Tugwell P, Knottnerus A. GRADE guidelines: a new series of articles in the Journal of Clinical Epidemiology. *J Clin Epidemiol* 2011;64:380-2.
2 Guyatt GH, Oxman AD, Kunz R, Falck-Ytter Y, Vist GE, Liberati A, et al. Going from evidence to recommendations. *BMJ* 2008;336:1049-51.
3 Guyatt GH, Oxman AD, Kunz R, Jaeschke R, Helfand M, Liberati A, et al. Incorporating considerations of resources use into grading recommendations. *BMJ* 2008;336:1170-3.
4 Guyatt GH, Oxman AD, Kunz R, Vist GE, Falck-Ytter Y, Schunemann HJ. What is "quality of evidence" and why is it important to clinicians? *BMJ* 2008;336:995-8.
5 Guyatt GH, Oxman AD, Vist GE, Kunz R, Falck-Ytter Y, Alonso-Coello P, et al. GRADE: an emerging consensus on rating quality of evidence and strength of recommendations. *BMJ* 2008;336:924-6.
6 Schunemann HJ, Oxman AD, Brozek J, Glasziou P, Jaeschke R, Vist GE, et al. Grading quality of evidence and strength of recommendations for diagnostic tests and strategies. *BMJ* 2008;336:1106-10.
7 You JJ, Singer DE, Howard PA, Lane DA, Eckman MH, Fang MC, et al. Antithrombotic therapy in atrial fibrillation: ACCP Evidence-Based Clinical Practice Guidelines, 9th edition. *Chest* 2012;141(2_suppl):e531S-75S.
8 Gage BF, van Walraven C, Pearce L, Hart RG, Koudstaal PJ, Boode BS, et al. Selecting patients with atrial fibrillation for anticoagulation: stroke risk stratification in patients taking aspirin. *Circulation* 2004;110:2287-92.
9 Singer DE, Chang Y, Fang MC, Borowsky LH, Pomernacki NK, Udaltsova N, et al. The net clinical benefit of warfarin anticoagulation in atrial fibrillation. *Ann Intern Med* 2009;151:297-305.
10 Hopewell S, Loudon K, Clarke MJ, Oxman AD, Dickersin K. Publication bias in clinical trials due to statistical significance or direction of trial results. *Cochrane Database Syst Rev* 2009;(1):MR000006.
11 Dickersin K, Min YI, Meinert CL. Factors influencing publication of research results. Follow-up of applications submitted to two institutional review boards. *JAMA* 1992;267:374-8.
12 Guyatt GH, Oxman AD, Montori V, Vist G, Kunz R, Brozek J, et al. GRADE guidelines: 5. Rating the quality of evidence—publication bias. *J Clin Epidemiol* 2011;64:1277-82.
13 Guyatt GH, Oxman AD, Kunz R, Brozek J, Alonso-Coello P, Rind D, et al. GRADE guidelines 6. Rating the quality of evidence—imprecision. *J Clin Epidemiol* 2011;64:1283-93.

STIMATES OF ABSOLUTE EFFECT

hen patients and clinicians are trading off desirable and undesirable consequences of an tervention they require estimates of absolute effect. For instance, patients with atrial fibrillation eed to trade off risk of strokes versus risk of major bleeding, and they need to know how any strokes anticoagulation will prevent, and how many strokes it will cause. This is best done y applying estimates of relative effect to estimates of baseline risk, such as by means of the HADS2 scoring system:

cenario 1

Patients with a CHADS2 score of 1 have a yearly risk of stroke of about 22 per 1000

The relative risk of stroke in patients receiving warfarin is 0.34

Therefore the risk of stroke in treated patients is 22×0.34 per 1000 = 7 per 1000

Thus, the absolute reduction in risk is 22−7 = 15 per 1000

cenario 2

Patients whose CHADS2 score is 2 have a yearly risk of stroke of about 45 per 1000

The relative risk of stroke in patients receiving warfarin is also 0.34 in this group

Therefore the risk of stroke in treated patients is 45×0.34 per 1000 = 15 per 1000

Thus, the absolute reduction in risk is 45−15 = 30 per 1000

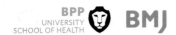

14   Bates SM, Greer IA, Veenstra D, Prabulos AM, Vandvik PO. Venous thromboembolism, thrombophilia, antithrombotic therapy, and pregnancy. ACCP Evidence-based Clinical Practice Guidelines, 9th Edition. *Chest* 2012;141(2_suppl):e691S-736S.

15   Mara M, Koryntova D, Rezabek K, Kapral A, Drbohlav P, Jirsova S, et al. [Thromboembolic complications in patients undergoing in vitro fertilization: retrospective clinical study]. *Ceska Gynekol* 2004;69:312-6.

16   Guyatt GH, Oxman AD, Kunz R, Woodcock J, Brozek J, Helfand M, et al. GRADE guidelines: 7. Rating the quality of evidence—inconsistency. *J Clin Epidemiol* 2011;64:1294-302.

17   Gould MK, Garcia DA, Wren SM, Karanicolas PJ, Arcelus JI, Heit JA, et al. Prevention of venous thromboembolism in non-orthopedic surgical patients: ACCP Evidence-based Clinical Practice Guideline, 9th Edition. *Chest* 2012;141(2_suppl):e227S-77S.

18   Danish SF, Burnett MG, Ong JG, Sonnad SS, Maloney-Wilensky E, Stein SC. Prophylaxis for deep venous thrombosis in craniotomy patients: a decision analysis. *Neurosurgery* 2005;56:1286-92, 92-4.

19   Guyatt GH, Oxman AD, Kunz R, Woodcock J, Brozek J, Helfand M, et al. GRADE guidelines: 8. Rating the quality of evidence—indirectness. *J Clin Epidemiol* 2011;64:1303-10.

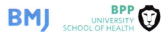

Value of composite reference standards in diagnostic research

Christiana A Naaktgeboren, PhD fellow, Loes C M Bertens, PhD fellow,
Maarten van Smeden, PhD fellow, Joris A H de Groot, assistant professor,
Karel G M Moons, professor, Johannes B Reitsma, associate professor

s Center for Health Sciences
Primary Care, University
cal Center Utrecht,
ersiteitsweg 100, 3584 CG
:ht, Netherlands

spondence to: C A
tgeboren c.naaktgeboren@
utrecht.nl

this as: *BMJ* 2013;347:f5605

10.1136/bmj.f5605

//www.bmj.com/content/347/
°5605

A common challenge in diagnostic studies is to obtain a correct final diagnosis in all participants. Ideally, a single error-free reference test, known as a gold standard, is used to determine the final diagnosis[1] and estimate the accuracy of the test or diagnostic model under evaluation. If the reference standard does not perfectly correspond to true target disease status, estimates of the accuracy of the test or model under study (index test), such as sensitivity, specificity, predictive values, or area under the curve, can be biased.[2] This is known as imperfect reference standard bias. One method to reduce this bias is to use a fixed rule to combine results of several imperfect tests into a composite reference standard.[3] When the combination of several component tests provides a better perspective on disease than any of the individual tests alone, accuracy estimates of the test under evaluation (the index test) will be less biased than if only one imperfect test is used as the reference standard. Comparing the index test against each component test separately and then averaging the accuracy estimates is not recommended; it is better to insightfully combine component tests together into a composite reference standard.

The hallmark of composite reference standards is that each combination of test results leads to a particular final diagnosis; in its simplest form, disease present or absent. For example, in a study on the accuracy of a rapid antigen test for detecting trichomoniasis, researchers decided against using the traditional gold standard of culture because it probably misses some cases.[4] As they believed that microscopy picks up additional true cases, they instead considered patients as diseased if either microscopy or culture results were abnormal. Table 1 gives further examples.

Although the choice of component tests and the rules used to combine them affects the estimates of accuracy of the test under study,[7] little guidance exists on how to develop and define a composite reference standard. Additionally, there is a lack of consensus in the way the term composite reference standard is used and reporting of results is generally poor. To address these problems,

ABSTRACT

Combining several tests is a common way to improve the final classification of disease status in diagnostic accuracy studies but is often used ambiguously. This article gives advice on proper use and reporting of composite reference standards

we provide an explanation of the methods for composite reference standards and make recommendations for development and reporting.

What is a composite reference standard?

A composite reference standard is a fixed rule used to make a final diagnosis based on the results of two or more tests, referred to as component tests. For each possible pattern of component test results (test profiles), a decision is made about whether it reflects presence or absence of the target disease.

Composite reference standards are appealing because of their similarity to clinical practice; they strongly resemble diagnostic rules that exist for several conditions, such as rheumatic fever and depression. Their main advantage is reproducibility of results, which is made possible by the transparency and consistency in the way that the final diagnosis is reached across participants. However, they also have disadvantages, the most glaring being the subjectivity introduced in the development of the rule.

The term "composite reference standard" is often loosely used as a catch-all term to describe any situation in which multiple reference tests are used to evaluate the accuracy of the index test. It is sometimes mistakenly used to describe differential verification, when different reference standards are used for different groups of participants (table 2).[8 9] It has also been used to describe discrepant analysis, a method in which the reference standard is re-run or re-evaluated, or a different reference standard is used, when the first one does not agree with the index test.[13] Both these approaches can lead to seriously biased estimates of accuracy and should be avoided whenever possible.

In the example in table 2 of a study on deep venous thrombosis differential verification was mislabelled as a composite reference standard. The reference standard for participants with a negative index test result was clinical follow-up while those with a positive result received the preferred reference standard, computed tomography.[11] If minor thromboembolisms that would have been picked up by computed tomography were missed during follow-up, the number of false negatives will be underestimated and the number of true negatives overestimated, thus biasing the accuracy estimates. Ethical or practical difficulties sometimes make it impossible to implement the same reference standard in all participants, but it is important that the term differential verification is used to describe such situations.

SUMMARY POINTS

A composite reference standard is a predefined rule that combines the results of multiple imperfect (component) tests in order to improve the classification of disease status in a diagnostic study

The term is often misused to describe differential verification, a situation in which different reference standards are used for different groups of participants

Different sets of component tests or different rules to combine the same component tests will lead to different estimates of accuracy for the test(s) under study

When using composite reference standards, it is important to prespecify and explain the rationale for the rule, report index test results for each combination of component tests, and explain how missing component test results are dealt with

Table 1 Examples of composite reference standards

Condition	Example	Rule for combination
Trichomoniasis[4]	"Samples were labeled as positive if the results of either mount microscopy or culture were positive… samples were labeled negative if both mount preparations and culture were negative"	Any positive rule
Typhoid fever[5]	"A composite reference standard of blood culture and polymerase chain reaction was used"	Any positive rule
Adherence to isoniazid preventive therapy for latent tuberculosis[6]	Adherence defined as .3 points when tests receive the following weights:	Heavier weights given to more accurate tests
	2 points for a positive urine isoniazid test result	
	1 point for patient observed taking tablets	
	1 for hospital records	
	1 point for patient self reporting	

Table 2 Examples of misuse of the term composite reference standard

Disease	Example	Explanation of misuse
Congenital heart defect[10]	"Pulse oximetry was performed prior to discharge and the results of this index test were compared with a composite reference standard (echocardiography, clinical follow-up and follow-up through interrogation of clinical databases)."	This is differential verification because some patients received an intensive clinical work-up while others were followed-up in clinical databases
Deep venous thrombosis[11]	"All patients were… diagnosed according to local protocols. Pulmonary embolism was confirmed or refuted on the basis of a composite reference standard, including spiral computed tomography and three months' follow-up."	This is differential verification because high risk patients had computed tomography whereas other patients were followed- up
Coronary artery stenosis[12]	"Diagnosis stenosis using composite findings from both [the index and the reference] tests as an enhanced reference standard . . . If a stenosis .50% had been seen on one [imaging test] but not on the other test, the observers closely re-evaluated the respective coronary artery segment showing discordant findings in order to confirm or revise their initial interpretation."	This is an example of discrepant analysis[13] in which the index test influences the reference standard result

Table 3 Effect of using different rules to produce composite reference standard on estimates of accuracy using example inspired by a study on the accuracy of rapid antigen detection test for trichomoniasis[4]

Result of component reference tests		Diagnosis with composite reference standard		Index test (rapid antigen detectiontest, n=100)	
Culture	Microscopy	Any positive rule*	All positive rule†	No with positive result	No with negative result
+	+	+	+	25	1
+	−	+	−	10	3
−	+	+	−	4	1
−	−	−	−	1	55

*Accuracy estimate using the any positive rule: sensitivity=(25+10+4)/((25+10+4)+(1+3+1))=0.89; specificity=55/(55+1)=0.98.

†Accuracy estimate using the all positive rule: sensitivity=25/(25+1)=0.96; specificity=(3+1+55)/((3+1+55)+(10+4+1))=0.8.

the same component tests and these component tests interpreted and combined in a fixed way for all patients

Developing a composite reference standard

As the choice of component tests and the rule for combin them strongly influences the accuracy of compo reference standards,[14] careful attention is required w developing the decision rule. Ideally, the combination test results and the corresponding final diagnosis shoul specified before the study to prevent data driven decisio However, if there is uncertainty about the best compo reference standard, a sensitivity analysis could be plan to see how sensitive the results are to the particular ch of tests or combination rule. It is also important that composite reference standard is clinically relevant. In o words, it should detect cases that will benefit from clir intervention rather than simply the presence of diseas For clinical situations when the true disease status car be defined the composite reference standard should ref the provisional working definition. Keeping diagno guidelines in mind and seeking advice from experts in field will help ensure that the chosen standard is clinic relevant and interpretable.

Defining rules to combine component tests

Two rules exist for combining component tests int composite reference standard. In the simplest scenaric two dichotomous component tests, participants could considered to have the disease if either test is indica of disease (any positive rule, also known as the "or" ru The alternative is that participants are considered to h the disease only if both tests detect disease (all positive "and" rule). If there are more than two component test combination of these two rules can be used.

Increasing the number of component tests will incre the number of participants categorised as diseased. If any positive rule is used, this will increase the sensitivity the composite reference standard (more diseased subje will be classified as diseased) but decrease its specifi (more non-diseased subjects will be classified as hav the disease). The reverse is true for the "all positive" r sensitivity of the composite reference standard decrea while specificity increases. Table 3 gives an example of h the choice of combination rule affects the accuracy of composite reference standard, which in turn affects accuracy estimates of the test under study.[2]

There is almost always a trade-off between sensitivity a specificity when considering alternative ways to comb component tests.[14] The exception is when a compon test in an "any positive" rule has perfect sensitiv which makes a composite reference standard with perf sensitivity, or when a component test in an "all positiv rule has perfect specificity, which makes a compos standard with perfect specificity.[3] Near perfect sensitiv or specificity of a component test is often the reason provided for the rule chosen.

Selection of component tests

Although it may be tempting to include numerous compon tests, the gain in sensitivity or specificity of the result composite reference standard decreases (and the clini interpretability may diminish) as more tests are add This is because additional tests may fail to provide n information. In the trichomoniasis example, if another t such as polymerase chain reaction amplification is add new true cases may be detected.[4] However, if yet anoth test is added, fewer additional true cases will be detec because fewer remained undetected. Eventually, all t

Table 2 also gives an example of discrepant analysis from an imaging study for coronary artery stenosis in which the reference standard results were re-evaluated when they did not agree with the index test results.[12] Such re-evaluation can only lead to increased agreement between index test and the reference standard, which in turn can only lead to overestimates of accuracy. Although discrepant analysis his highly discouraged, situations in which the reference standard is repeated or a different reference standard is applied in those patients where the index test and first reference standard disagree, should be termed discrepant analysis.

To avoid confusion we recommend using the term composite reference standard exclusively for situations in which, by design, all patients are intended to receive

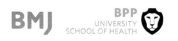

le 4 Use of a composite reference standard to determine different categories of diagnosis turberculosis[17]

al diagnosis	Individual tests				
	Acid fast bacilli smear	Culture	Radiology	Histology	Follow-up
nfirmed	+/-	+	+/-	+/-	+
bable	+/-	-	+	+	+
	+/-	-	+		+
	+/-	-	-	+	+
ssible	+/-	-	-	-	+
erculosis	-	-	-	-	-

le 5 Template for reporting results when using a composite reference standard

Composite reference standard				Index test*	
Test 1	Test 2	Test 3	Final diagnosis	No with positive result	No with negative result
+	+	+	+	p_1	n_1
+	+	-	+ or -	p_2	n_2
+	-	+	+ or -	p_3	n_3
+	-	-	+ or -	p_4	n_4
-	+	+	+ or -	p_5	n_5
-	+	-	+ or -	p_6	n_6
-	-	+	+ or -	p_7	n_7
-	-	-	-	p_8	n_8

cases are detected and additional tests will only result in false positive results, thus decreasing the specificity of the composite reference standard.

Multiple tests will be useful only if the component tests catch each other's mistakes. For example, in a group of patients who truly have trichomoniasis, if microscopy identifies disease in the same participants as culture does, microscopy does not add any information and therefore the sensitivity of the composite reference standard will not be higher than that of culture alone.[2] When component tests make the same classifications in truly diseased or non-diseased patients more or less often than is expected by chance alone, this is referred to as conditional dependence.

In some cases, conditional dependence can be avoided or reduced by choosing component tests that look at different biological aspects of the disease.[16] To avoid causing the tests to make the same mistakes, you should consider blinding the observer of each component test to the results of the other component tests if knowledge of these other test results can influence interpretation.

Extensions to the basic composite reference standard
The basic composite reference standard categorises patients simply as diseased or non-diseased. However, multiple disease categories can also be defined, such as subtypes, stages, or degree of certainty of disease. An example is a study on tuberculosis in which people were categorised into one of four levels of disease certainty (table 4).[17]

The basic composite reference standard gives equal weight to all tests, but in clinical practice tests carry different weights. The relative importance of the component tests can be incorporated by assigning weights. For example, in the assessment of adherence to isoniazid treatment for latent tuberculosis in table 1, the most reliable test was given twice the weight of the other tests.[6]

Missing values on component tests
As with all diagnostic accuracy studies, results may be biased when not all participants receive the intended reference standard.[8] Careful attention needs to be paid to

missing values in component tests. For example, if the "any positive" rule is used and the result of component test 1 is positive, we can conclude that a patient is diseased without knowing the result of component test 2. For efficiency, researchers might consider skipping the second test in participants whose first test result is positive.[3][18] However, if component test 1 is negative, component test 2 becomes necessary for determining the diagnosis.

When a result is missing from a component test that must be present under the combination rules, the composite reference standard is also missing. This may affect the accuracy estimates of the index test and mathematical methods should be used to tentatively correct for this bias.[19]

Reporting guidelines
Complete and accurate reporting of the reference standard procedure is critical to allow readers to judge the potential risk of bias in accuracy estimates. This is especially important for systematic reviews of diagnostic tests. The validity of comparing accuracy estimates between studies and pooling of estimates across studies is challenged when studies use different reference standards or when reference standards are poorly defined or reported.[20][21] We therefore recommend that in addition to using current reporting guidelines,[22] authors of diagnostic accuracy studies should include the following details about studies with composite reference standards:

- The rationale behind the selection of component tests and the combination rule
- The corresponding final diagnosis for each combination of test results
- Whether component test results were missing and and whether this resulted in a missing composite reference standard
- The number of participants with each combination of test results. For continuous tests, this information should at least be provided for the optimal or most common cut-off point.

Table 5 gives a template for reporting. The availability of all of the above information will allow studies using composite reference standards to be compared with those using only one of the component tests as the reference standard.

Conclusions and recommendations
Combining multiple tests to define a target disease status rather than using a single imperfect test is a transparent and reproducible method for dealing with the common problem of imperfect reference standard bias. Although composite reference standards may reduce the amount of such bias, they cannot completely eliminate it because it is unlikely that a combination of imperfect tests will produce a composite standard with perfect sensitivity and specificity.

Other methods for dealing with bias resulting from imperfect reference standards are panel diagnosis and latent class analysis.[1][3] In panel diagnosis, multiple experts review relevant patient characteristics, test results, and sometimes follow-up information before coming to a consensus about the final diagnosis in each patient. Latent class analysis estimates accuracy by assuming that true disease status is unobservable and relating the results of multiple tests to it in a statistical model.[3][23] The choice of method to deal with imperfect reference standard bias will probably depend on the type, number, and accuracy of the pieces of diagnostic information available in a particular study. Results from all three methods could be presented to strengthen their

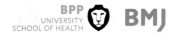

face validity. Researchers who use a composite reference standard can improve the transparency and reproducibility of their results by following our recommendations on reporting.

Contributors: All authors participated in the conception and design of the article, worked on the drafting of the article and revising it critically for important intellectual content, and have approved the final version to be published. CAN had the idea for the article, performed the literature search, and wrote the article. JBR is the guarantor.

Competing interests: All authors read and understood the BMJ policy on declaration of interests and declare financial support from Netherlands Organization for Scientific Research (project 918.10.615).

Provenance and peer review: Not commissioned; externally peer reviewed.

1   Rutjes AW, Reitsma JB, Coomarasamy A, Khan KS, Bossuyt PM. Evaluation of diagnostic tests when there is no gold standard. A review of methods. *Health Technol Assess* 2007;11:iii, ix-51.
2   Walter SD, Macaskill P, Lord SJ, Irwig L. Effect of dependent errors in the assessment of diagnostic or screening test accuracy when the reference standard is imperfect. *Stat Med* 2012;31:1129-38.
3   Alonzo TA, Pepe MS. Using a combination of reference tests to assess the accuracy of a new diagnostic test. *Stat Med* 1999;18:2987-3003.
4   Hegazy MM, El-Tantawy NL, Soliman MM, El-Sadeek ES, El-Nagar HS. Performance of rapid immunochromatographic assay in the diagnosis of Trichomoniasis vaginalis. *Diagn Microbiol Infect Dis* 2012;74:49-53.
5   Siba V, Horwood PF, Vanuga K, Wapling J, Sehuko R, Siba PM, et al. Evaluation of serological diagnostic tests for typhoid fever in Papua New Guinea using a composite reference standard. *Clin Vaccine Immunol* 2012;19:1833-7.
6   Nicolau I, Tian L, Menzies D, Ostiguy G, Pai M. Point-of-care urine tests for smoking status and isoniazid treatment monitoring in adult patients. *PLoS One* 2012;7:e45913.
7   Hadgu A, Dendukuri N, Wang L. Evaluation of screening tests for detecting Chlamydia trachomatis: bias associated with the patient-infected-status algorithm. *Epidemiology* 2012;23:72-82.
8   De Groot JA, Bossuyt PM, Reitsma JB, Rutjes AW, Dendukuri N, Janssen KJ, et al. Verification problems in diagnostic accuracy studies: consequences and solutions. *BMJ* 2011;343:d4770.
9   Naaktgeboren CA, de Groot JAH, van Smeeden M, Moons KGM, Reitsma JB. Evaluating diagnostic accuracy in the face of multiple reference standards. *Ann Intern Med* 2013;159:195-202.
10 Ewer AK, Furmston AT, Middleton LJ, Deeks JJ, Daniels JP, Pattison HM, et al. Pulse oximetry as a screening test for congenital heart defects in newborn infants: a test accuracy study with evaluation of acceptability and cost-effectiveness. *Health Technol Assess* 2012;16:v-184.
11 Geersing GJ, Erkens PM, Lucassen WA, Buller HR, Cate HT, Hoes AW, et al. Safe exclusion of pulmonary embolism using the Wells rule and qualitative D-dimer testing in primary care: prospective cohort study. *BMJ* 2012;345:e6564.
12 Kerl JM, Schoepf UJ, Zwerner PL, Bauer RW, Abro JA, Thilo C, et al. Accuracy of coronary artery stenosis detection with CT versus conventional coronary angiography compared with composite findings from both tests as an enhanced reference standard. *Eur Radiol* 2011;21:1895-903.
13 Hadgu A. The discrepancy in discrepant analysis. *Lancet* 1996;348:592-3.
14 Macaskill P, Walter SD, Irwig L, Franco EL. Assessing the gain in diagnostic performance when combining two diagnostic tests. *Stat Med* 2002;21:2527-46.
15 Lord SJ, Staub LP, Bossuyt PM, Irwig LM. Target practice: choosing target conditions for test accuracy studies that are relevant to clinical practice. *BMJ* 2011;343:d4684.
16 Gardner IA, Stryhn H, Lind P, Collins MT. Conditional dependence between tests affects the diagnosis and surveillance of animal diseases. *Prev Vet Med* 2000;45:107-22.
17 Vadwai V, Boehme C, Nabeta P, Shetty A, Alland D, Rodrigues C. Xpert MTB/RIF: a new pillar in diagnosis of extrapulmonary tuberculosis? *J Clin Microbiol* 2011;49:2540-5.
18 Hilden J. Boolean algebra, Boolean nodes. In: Kattan M, Cowen ME, eds. Encyclopedia of medical decision making. 1st ed. Sage, 2009:94-8.
19 De Groot JA, Janssen KJ, Zwinderman AH, Bossuyt PM, Reitsma JB, Moons KG. Correcting for partial verification bias: a comparison of methods. *Ann Epidemiol* 2011;21:139-48.
20 Whiting PF, Rutjes AW, Westwood ME, Mallett S, Deeks JJ, Reitsma JB, et al. QUADAS-2: a revised tool for the quality assessment of diagnostic accuracy studies. *Ann Intern Med* 2011;155:529-36.
21 Lijmer JG, Bossuyt PM, Heisterkamp SH. Exploring sources of heterogeneity in systematic reviews of diagnostic tests. *Stat Med* 2002;21:1525-37.
22 Bossuyt PM, Reitsma JB, Bruns DE, Gatsonis CA, Glasziou PP, Irwig LM, et al. Towards complete and accurate reporting of studies of diagnostic accuracy: the STARD initiative. *Fam Pract* 2004;21:4-10.
23 Pepe MS, Janes H. Insights into latent class analysis of diagnostic test performance. *Biostatistics* 2007;8:474-84.

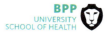

Diagnostic accuracy studies: how to report and analyse inconclusive test results

Bethany Shinkins, DPhil student in primary healthcare, Matthew Thompson, clinical reader in primary healthcare, Susan Mallett, senior medical statistician, Rafael Perera, director of statistics

ersity of Oxford, Department
imary Care Health Sciences,
liffe Observatory Quarter,
rd OX2 6GG, UK

espondence to: B Shinkins
any.shinkins@phc.ox.ac.uk

this as: BMJ 2013;346:f2778

10.1136/bmj.f2778

/www.bmj.com/content/346/
2778

The results of studies on diagnostic test accuracy are often reported as a 2×2 classification matrix, in which test results are presented as a dichotomy and a reference standard is used to categorise individuals as with or without disease. This facilitates the calculation of many popular statistics used to summarise the discriminatory performance of tests (such as sensitivity and specificity, positive and negative likelihood ratios, and positive and negative predictive values). Restricting test results to be either positive or negative, however, fails to represent the reality of how they are used in clinical practice[1] ; in many cases, the results from a given diagnostic test do not exclusively fall into these "positive" and "negative" categories.

Although most test results provide useful information for diagnostic decision making, there is often a subset of results that are relatively uninformative and lead to an "inconclusive" diagnostic outcome. For example, the "normal" range on a standard biomarker is typically based on statistics that try to minimise the number of false classifications. As most biomarkers are far from perfect discriminators, however, results that fall close to the lower and upper limits of "normality" provide minimal information about the disease status of the patient and are therefore "inconclusive." In most cases inconclusive test results require extra attention from clinicians, such as repeating the test or using more costly (in terms of invasiveness, time, and expense) diagnostic tools. All of these outcomes, coupled with the inevitable delay in diagnosis and clinical decision making, directly affect patient care.

In this paper we have focused on clinical scenarios in which there are two disease categories—disease present and disease absent—and discuss the reporting and analysis of inconclusive results produced by a single index test—that is, the diagnostic test under evaluation. Although this is a common scenario in research on diagnostic test accuracy, this is often a simplification of the actual clinical question. In practice, diagnostic tests are often used to distinguish between multiple diseases or different levels of severity, such as different staging in diagnosis of cancer. Additionally,

ABSTRACT

Failure to report inconclusive test results can lead to misleading conclusions regarding the accuracy and clinical usefulness of a diagnostic tool. We show that these results are often overlooked in research on test accuracy and provide guidance on suitable approaches to reporting and analysing these problematic results.

the diagnostic process might involve a pathway of multiple tests rather than a single test.

Inconsistent reporting of inconclusive test results in research on diagnostic accuracy

We wanted to explore whether inconclusive results are consistently reported in diagnostic accuracy research. The STARD (STAndards for the Reporting of Diagnostic accuracy studies) statement—a reporting guideline encouraging high quality reporting of diagnostic accuracy studies—recommends that authors "report how indeterminate results, missing responses and outliers of the index tests are handled."[2] The full STARD guidance expands on this statement, advocating the reporting of "uninterpretable, indeterminate, and intermediate results" (item 22). We assessed systematic reviews to evaluate how well primary diagnostic accuracy studies adhere to this recommendation (box).

Based on 1156 primary studies included in 22 systematic reviews (published between 2005 and 2011), we found that only a third (35%) of studies reported the presence or absence of inconclusive results adequately, showing that these results are not consistently reported in diagnostic accuracy research.[3 4 5 6 7 8 9 10 11 12 13 14 15 16 17 18 19 20 21 22 23 24] The wide variation in the proportion of studies that were adherent between reviews could indicate that there was some reviewer subjectivity in the interpretation of the STARD item and how they defined adherence. As the reviews assessed studies based on all the STARD items (25 in total), there was little discussion by the authors about the specific criteria used to define "adherence" to each item, though most of the systematic reviews used more than one reviewer to assess reporting quality.

QUADAS—a tool for assessing the quality of diagnostic accuracy studies included in systematic reviews—asks reviewers to check that "uninterpretable, indeterminate or intermediate test results" are reported.[25] In a recent evaluation of QUADAS, authors of Cochrane reviews reported that this recommendation was difficult to apply because of confusion about the applicability to particular diagnostic tests. They also noted important issues surrounding reliability between raters.[26]

These findings support the need to clarify the importance of inconclusive results and provide clear guidance to researchers on how to handle these results when reporting and analysing diagnostic accuracy studies.

SUMMARY POINTS

Reporting tips

Report the causes and frequencies of any uninterpretable or missing results, broken down by the reference standard

Report all valid inconclusive results on their original scale (that is, before any grouping of results), again broken down by the reference standard

For tests of a continuous scale or an ordinal scale with lots of categories, plots should be used

Analysis tips

The accuracy of an index test should be analysed in line with how the test will be used in clinical practice

If valid inconclusive results are excluded from analyses, accuracy statistics should be reported when the inconclusive results are included as a secondary (sensitivity) analysis

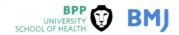

Table 1 Clinical examples of uninterpretable results

Diagnostic scenario	Examples of uninterpretable test results
Cervical smear test for evidence of cervical cancer	No endocervical cells could be observed, possibly because of inflammation or poor sampling technique[31]
Two dimensional echocardiography for determining aortic valve structure	Echocardiogram is uninterpretable because of heavy calcification and/or poor image quality[30]
Urine culture	Contaminated with bacterial overgrowth in sample delayed in transport to laboratory
Ultrasonography	Inability to visualise appendix with ultrasonography because of retrocaecal position

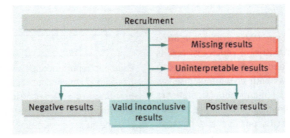

Fig 1 Flowchart of index test results distinguishing between valid and invalid inconclusive index test results

Defining inconclusive results

Types of inconclusive test results
Simel and colleagues outlined three main types of "non-positive, non-negative" results[27]:

- Uninterpretable results: those that "do not meet the minimum criteria constituting an adequate test"

- Intermediate test results: those that "confer a likelihood ratio for disease that is more than that conferred by a negative result, but less than that of a positive test"

- Indeterminate test results: those that add no additional diagnostic information to the original probability of disease. In technical terms, this is a test result with a likelihood ratio of about 1, meaning that knowledge of the test result does not alter the probability of disease.

In reported studies, however, the distinction between the different types of results is often lost, and the terms are used interchangeably—see, for example, the studies by Kamath and colleagues,[28] Glaser and colleagues,[29] and Ayad and colleagues.[30] We have provided some clarity on methods for reporting and analysing inconclusive index test results in diagnostic accuracy studies. To facilitate this, we firstly differentiated between inconclusive results that are invalid (that is, the key diagnostic feature is uninterpretable or the actual result is missing) and those that are valid (that is, where an adequate test result has been obtained, but the result is not clearly positive or negative). This distinction affects how inconclusive test results should be reported and analysed (fig 1).

Invalid inconclusive results

Uninterpretable and missing index test results
A test result is "uninterpretable" when the key diagnostic feature of the result is either missing, obstructed, or of questionable validity because of an inadequate test procedure (table 1 shows some clinical examples). In some cases, uninterpretable results occur because the test was not conducted to an acceptable standard (such as a cervical smear test carried out with poor sampling technique or a contaminated urine culture), and in others it could be because a clinical feature of the patient hampers the

ADHERENCE TO STARD

- **Methods** We searched Embase and Medline using the term "STARD" [All fields] to identify systematic reviews assessin adherence to the STARD statement.

- **Results** Twenty two systematic reviews met the inclusion criteria, comprising 1156 primary diagnostic accuracy studies. Based on reported adherence in the systematic reviews, only 35% (400/1156) of diagnostic accuracy studies explicitly reported uninterpretable, indeterminate, intermediate, and missing results. There was a wide variation in adherence across systematic reviews (range 0-66%), indicating that there was inconsistency in the quality of reporting in different clinical areas and/or the reviewers' interpretation of the STARD statement.

- **Conclusion** Inconclusive results in diagnostic accuracy studies are not consistently reported, with around a third studies fully complying with item 22 of the STARD stateme (see appendix 1 and 2 for full details of methods and table of results).

interpretation of the test (such as an uninterpretable cerv smear because of concurrent infection or a retrocaec positioned appendix resulting in difficult visualisa on ultrasonography). Invalid inconclusive test results caused by an intrinsic property of the test (an objec quality) rather than the relative importance of false posi and false negative results. In contrast, missing results oc when a patient should have been included in a study no test result is recorded. Missing results are often hand in a similar way to uninterpretable results.

In the presence of uninterpretable and missing resu it is vital to consider the underlying reasons.[32] If occurrence of the result is not influenced by the prese or absence of disease, such as the accidental contamina of a urine culture with skin bacteria, then the test can o simply be repeated. In some cases, however, the prese of an uninterpretable result can be informative—it increa or decreases the probability of disease—despite not be categorised as a positive or negative result.[32] For exam by exploring the possible causes of uninterpretable res in the evaluation of the accuracy of two dimensic transthoracic echocardiography for determining aortic va structure, Ayad and colleagues identified a relation betw the valve weight (from calcification) and whether the im could be interpreted.[30]

Valid inconclusive results

The ways in which valid inconclusive results should reported and analysed depends on the measurement s of the test: results can be continuous, categorical, or ord in nature.

Continuous inconclusive index test results
Inconclusive results can occur for index tests measu on a continuous test scale (such as biochemical assa (table 2 gives examples). They typically lie in the ra of values where the distributions of abnormal values normal values overlap (fig 2), although the degree to wh they encompass this region of uncertainty depends on relative implications of false positive and false negative outcomes. These results are valid index test results, the same result should be obtained if the test is repea (putting aside random measurement error and tempe changes).

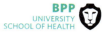

Table 2 Clinical examples of continuous inconclusive index test results

Diagnostic scenario	Examples of continuous inconclusive test results
Brain natriuretic peptide (BNP) for diagnosis of heart failure in patients with acute dyspnoea[33]	No heart failure: 0-167 ng/L; inconclusive result: 167-462 ng/L; heart failure: 462-5000 ng/L
Procalcitonin for diagnosis of early onset neonatal sepsis[34]	No sepsis: <0.5 μg/L; inconclusive result: 0.5-20 μg/L; sepsis: >20 μg/L
Management of patients with diabetes in primary care with chronic kidney disease using eGFR	Monitor annually: eGFR ≥60; inconclusive result: eGFR 30-59; refer: eGFR <30
eGFR=estimated glomerular filtration rate.	

eGFR=estimated glomerular filtration rate.

Table 3 Clinical examples of categorical and ordinal inconclusive index test results

Diagnostic scenario	Examples of categorical and ordinal inconclusive test results
Imaging for cancer staging	Detected lesion that cannot be characterised as metastatic or non-metastatic based on imaging scan[35]
Thyroid nodule evaluation with fine needle aspiration biopsy	Cytological features that are overlapping and cannot clearly be distinguished as benign or malignant[36]
Western blot test for HIV infection	Tests that have one or more protein bands but do not meet criteria for positive result[37]
Ordinal: General Health Questionnaire-12 screening tool for mental health disorders in primary care	Low chance of mental disorder: scores <4; intermediate chance of mental disorder: scores 4-6; high chance of mental disorder: scores 7-12[38]

Table 4 Proposed 3×2 classification table, with allowance for reporting of valid inconclusive test results

Test result	Disease status	
	Disease present	Disease absent
Positive	True positive	False positive
Valid inconclusive	Disease absent but valid inconclusive result	Disease present but valid inconclusive result
Negative	False negative	True negative

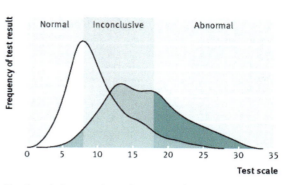

Fig 2 Inconclusive range for continuous test where two underlying distributions of test results overlap

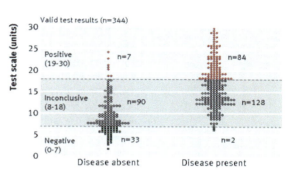

Fig 3 Dot plot for continuous index test with thresholds (hypothetical data)

Categorical/ordinal inconclusive index test results

Inconclusive results can also occur when test results are categorised into groups according to characteristics rather than continuous values. For categorical tests, inconclusive results can occur when some results cannot be placed in either the positive or negative categories (table 3 gives examples). For ordinal tests (such as symptom scores), there are often multiple ordered categories of result, where the middle category/categories do not provide sufficient evidence regarding the presence or absence of disease. As with a continuous inconclusive result, categorical and ordinal inconclusive results are valid test outcomes, and repeating the test should produce another inconclusive result (barring variability within the patient and progression of disease over time).

How to report inconclusive results

Valid inconclusive results

To improve reporting of inconclusive results, the standard 2×2 classification matrix can be extended to a 3×2 matrix.[1][27] Simel and colleagues proposed that intermediate, indeterminate, and uninterpretable results should be grouped together to form a row of "uncertain" or "inconclusive" results.[27] We propose that the classification table should be limited to valid test results (table 4).

Continuous inconclusive test results

For index tests on a continuous test scale, "rule in" and "rule out" thresholds can be selected, leaving a range of valid inconclusive test values.[39] In some cases, a richer interpretation of accuracy is required and the test scale is partitioned into multiple (more than three) categories. Either way, the number of patients with positive and negative test results for a disease in each category should be cross tabulated, with extra rows to account for any additional categories. A full description of how and when

thresholds have been selected should be included in the methods section.

In addition to the classification table, it is essential to show the distribution of the raw test results, stratified by disease status (determined by the reference standard). Possible graphical options include paired histograms, dot plots, or cumulative distribution graphs. Addition of the thresholds and colour coding to plots can help readers understand where cut offs have been placed (fig 3).

Categorical/ordinal inconclusive test results

For categorical and ordinal index tests, the number of patients in each category should be reported and broken down by presence or absence of the target condition. For ordinal tests with a large number of categories (such as questionnaire scores), it might be sensible to group some of the categories for the classification table. If this is the case, it is still important to report a cross tabulation or plot of the frequencies in each original category and explain how the category groupings were determined.

Invalid inconclusive results

Reporting uninterpretable and missing inconclusive test results

Although uninterpretable and missing results are often not directly related to test accuracy, they are still an essential consideration in the evaluation of the overall clinical utility of the test. Uninterpretable and missing results should be reported separately from the cross tabulation of valid results by disease status, in addition to any known underlying causes, so that the reader can assess whether they hold any diagnostic value. Clear reporting and discussion of whether these results are related to the patient's disease status, the presence of an alternative target condition, or assumed to be unrelated to patient health enables transparency in how these results should be handled.

Table 5 Classification table of CT urography results[40]

Result	Presence of bladder cancer	
	Cancer present	Cancer absent
Positive	130	1
Valid inconclusive	10	101
Negative	8	497

The STARD statement recommends that a flowchart of participants at each stage of the study is reported.[2] Inclusion of all inconclusive results in this chart greatly enhances the transparency of test performance (see fig 4 for an example). The number of participants meeting the eligibility criteria (intention to diagnose) should feature in the flow diagram. Supplementary information such as the causes of uninterpretable or missing results should be reported separately.

How to analyse inconclusive test results

Inconclusive results can be difficult to analyse given that many statistics used to summarise the accuracy of diagnostic tests require the test results to be split into two groups. There is no single "optimal" approach to analysing inconclusive results; diagnostic accuracy should always be analysed in line with how the test will be used in clinical practice.

When exploring different testing strategies for the diagnosis of bladder cancer, Blick and colleagues reported both invalid (uninterpretable) and valid inconclusive results from computed tomography urography.[40] They excluded from the analyses the uninterpretable results that were caused by technical failures (five of 747) as they were found to be unrelated to disease status, but the causes and frequencies of these technical failures were still fully reported. If the occurrence of uninterpretable results had been found to be associated with the presence or absence of bladder cancer, exclusion of these results might not have been appropriate.

For valid inconclusive results, there are three common approaches to analysing categorical and ordinal inconclusive results. To illustrate these methods, we have used results from Blick's study assessing the accuracy of computed tomography (CT) urography for diagnosing bladder cancer (table 5).[40] It is important to note that, although not reported in this section for brevity, confidence intervals are a vital consideration in the interpretation of accuracy statistics. Methods for analysis of tests on continuous scales with valid inconclusive results are discussed at the end of this section.

Scenario 1: Exclude valid inconclusive results completely
An unfortunately common approach to dealing with this type of valid but inconclusive result is to exclude them completely from all analyses.[27] There are few instances where this can be justified, and this approach can lead to overstated summary statistics and promotion of suboptim test strategies.

For the CT urography data,[40] if the valid inconclusi results (15% of patient data) had simply been exclud this would have resulted in a sensitivity and specificity 94% and 100% and a positive and negative predictive val of 99% and 98%, respectively. This would have artificia inflated the accuracy of the test to near perfect accura resulting in flawed interpretation.

Scenario 2: Exclude valid inconclusive results from binary statistics but report an additional summary statistic that accounts for them

Another method is to exclude valid inconclusive resu from accuracy statistics such as sensitivity and specifici but report an additional statistic that takes into account t presence of inconclusive results.

One example is the percentage of the test results includ in the calculation of the binary summary statistics, oft referred to as the "test yield."[27] If the test yield is mu below 100%, then the reader should be aware that te results have been excluded. In the bladder cancer study, t "test yield" statistic would have been 85% if the 111 va inconclusive results had been wrongly excluded.

An alternative is to provide the number of corre classifications as a percentage of the total number of te results (including valid inconclusive test results), known "effectiveness."[41] If the percentage of valid inconclusi results is large, the effectiveness of the test will provi a more conservative estimate than the commonly us but flawed "accuracy" statistic that excludes inconclusi results. The "effectiveness" of CT urography in the bladd cancer example including valid inconclusive results is 84 compared with 99% if the inconclusive results are exclude

The risk of simply providing an additional statistic account for inconclusive results is that readers might strugg to interpret such unfamiliar statistics and interpret only t more popular accuracy measures, such as sensitivity a specificity. Furthermore, these additional statistics are n typically included in meta-analyses, where usually only t sensitivity and specificity are analysed.

Scenario 3: Group valid inconclusive results with positive c negative results
One way of overcoming the issue of analysing va inconclusive results is to group them with either t positive or negative results, depending on how the patients would be treated in the clinical context. In the evaluation of different roles for CT urography in diagnosis bladder cancer, Blick and colleagues assessed accuracy CT urography as a replacement test for flexible cystosco In this context, because of the high clinical cost of missi a cancer diagnosis, inconclusive CT urography resu should be grouped with positive results, as clinically the patients would still have to undergo rigid cystoscopy.[40] a replacement test, CT urography has a sensitivity a specificity of 95% and 83% and a positive and negati predictive value of 58% and 98%, respectively. The positi predictive value is notably lower when valid inconclusi results are included in the analyses (58% v 99%), whi gives a much more realistic representation of the tr accuracy of the test.

Grouping valid inconclusive results with either the positi or negative test results can cause considerable differenc in the summaries of test performance.[27][32][42] Often this reported as a secondary (or sensitivity) analysis. Subh

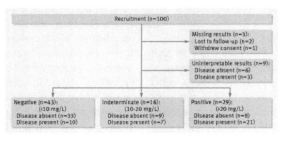

Fig Example flowchart for reporting results from diagnostic accuracy study of quantitative index test (hypothetical data)

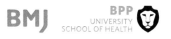

and colleagues adopted this approach when they assessed the accuracy of magnetic resonance imaging to diagnose meniscal tears,[43] showing that the specificity of the five point grading scale dropped from 94% to 47% depending on which grades were considered positive. This makes the discriminatory performance of the test completely transparent to the reader.

Analysis of continuous inconclusive test results

Any categorisation of a continuous test scale results in a loss of information.[44][45] The dichotomisation of continuous test scales, however, has become commonplace to make it easier for clinicians to interpret test results in the context of the clinical problem. For multivariate diagnostic prediction models, it has been strongly argued that the categorisation of continuous test scales (which are included as predictors in the model) is simply a waste of information because the predicted probability of disease is the key diagnostic outcome.[45] For the interpretation of results from a single continuous diagnostic test, however, some categorisation is usually helpful.

Several studies have found that moving away from the dichotomous partition of quantitative test scales and identifying intermediate range(s) of test results has enabled a better understanding of the diagnostic accuracy potential of a test.[34][46] Multi-level or stratum specific likelihood ratios have been proposed as a preferable way of summarising the performance of tests on a quantitative test scale. Allowance for multiple ranges of a test result retains more diagnostic information,[38][47][48][49] and the results are less susceptible to spectrum bias.[50]

Conclusion

Reporting and analysis of inconclusive test results have been relatively neglected in diagnostic accuracy studies. We encourage researchers and clinicians to clearly report all inconclusive results, broken down by the reference standard when possible. Complete transparency regarding the handling of inconclusive results in the analysis phase is essential for the reader to understand how key summary statistics have been derived. A well reported diagnostic accuracy study will allow readers to fully understand if and how inconclusive results were incorporated into analyses and provide them with sufficient information to recalculate key statistics if they disagree with the approach adopted by the author.

We thank Johannes Reitsma, who reviewed our first manuscript, which contributed extensively to the format and content of the final paper. We also thank Richard Mayon-White for his guidance in developing the ideas underlying this paper.

Contributors: BS initiated the study as part of her DPhil project. All co-authors contributed to the drafting of the manuscript. BS is guarantor.

Funding: BS is funded by the National School for Primary Care Research Capacity Building Award. MT, RP, and SM receive funding by the National Institute for Health Research (NIHR) under its programme grants for applied research funding scheme (RP-PG-0407-10347 and RP-PG-0407-10338). This paper presents independent research funded by the National Institute for Health Research (NIHR). The views expressed in this paper are those of the authors and not necessarily those of the NHS, the NIHR or the Department of Health

Competing interests: All authors have completed the ICMJE uniform disclosure form at www.icmje.org/coi_disclosure.pdf (available on request from the corresponding author) and declare: no support from any organisation for the submitted work; no financial relationships with any organisations that might have an interest in the submitted work in the previous three years; no other relationships or activities that could appear to have influenced the submitted work.

Provenance and peer review: Not commissioned; externally peer reviewed.

1 Feinstein AR. The inadequacy of binary models for the clinical reality of three-zone diagnostic decisions. *J Clin Epidemiol* 1990;43:109-13.

2 Bossuyt PM, Reitsma JB. The STARD initiative. *Lancet* 2003;361:71.

3 Areia M, Soares M, Dinis-Ribeiro M. Quality reporting of endoscopic diagnostic studies in gastrointestinal journals: Where do we stand on the use of the STARD and CONSORT statements? *Endoscopy* 2010;42:138-47.

4 Coppus SFPJ, van der Veen F, Bossuyt PMM, Mol BWJ. Quality of reporting of test accuracy studies in reproductive medicine: impact of the Standards for Reporting of Diagnostic Accuracy (STARD) initiative. *Fertil Steril* 2006;86:1321-9.

5 Fontela PS, Pai NP, Schiller I, Dendukuri N, Ramsay A, Pai M. Quality and reporting of diagnostic accuracy studies in TB, HIV and malaria: evaluation using QUADAS and STARD standards. *PlsOne* 2009;4:e7753.

6 Freeman K, Szczepura A, Osipenko L. Non-invasive fetal RHD genotyping tests: a systematic review of the quality of reporting of diagnostic accuracy in published studies. *Eur J Obstet Gynecol Reprod Biol* 2009;142:91-8.

7 Hing W, White S, Reid D, Marshall R. Validity of the McMurray's test and modified versions of the test: a systematic literature review. *J Man Manip Ther* 2009;17:22-35.

8 Jahromi AS, Cina CS, Liu Y, Clase CM. Sensitivity and specificity of color duplex ultrasound measurement in the estimation of internal carotid artery stenosis: a systematic review and meta-analysis. *J Vasc Surg* 2005;41:962-72.

9 Johnson ZK, Siddiqui MAR, Azuara-Blanco A. The quality of reporting of diagnostic accuracy studies of optical coherence tomography in glaucoma. *Ophthalmology* 2007;114:1607-12.

10 Krzych LJ, Liszka L. No improvement in studies reporting the diagnostic accuracy of B-type natriuretic peptide. *Med Sci Mon* 2009;15:5-14.

11 Legare F, Moher D, Elwyn G, LeBlanc A, Gravel K. Instruments to assess the perception of physicians in the decision-making process of specific clinical encounters: a systematic review. *BMC Med Inform Decis Mak* 2007;7:30.

12 Lumbreras B, Jarrin I, Hernandez Aguado I. Evaluation of the research methodology in genetic, molecular and proteomic tests. *Gaceta Sanitaria* 2006;20:368-73

13 Mahoney J, Ellison J. Assessing the quality of glucose monitor studies: a critical evaluation of published reports. *Clin Chem* 2007;53:1122-8.

14 Miller E, Roposch A, Uleryk E, Doria AS. Juvenile idiopathic arthritis of peripheral joints. Quality of reporting of diagnostic accuracy of conventional MRI1. *Acad Radiol* 2009;16:739-57.

15 Paranjothy B, Shunmugam M, Azuara-Blanco A. The quality of reporting of diagnostic accuracy studies in glaucoma using scanning laser polarimetry. *J Glaucoma* 2007;16:670-5.

16 Perry AE, Marandos R, Coulton S, Johnson M. Screening tools assessing risk of suicide and self-harm in adult offenders: a systematic review. *Int J Offender Ther Comp Criminol* 2010;54:803-28.

17 Roposch A, Moreau NM, Uleryk E, Doria AS. Developmental dysplasia of the hip: quality of reporting of diagnostic accuracy for US. *Radiology* 2006;241:854-60.

18 Selman TJ, Khan KS, Mann CH. An evidence-based approach to test accuracy studies in gynecologic oncology: the 'STARD' checklist. *Gynecol Oncol* 2005;96:575-8.

19 Selman TJ, Morris RK, Zamora J, Khan KS. The quality of reporting of primary test accuracy studies in obstetrics and gynaecology: application of the STARD criteria. *BMC Women's Health* 2011;11:8.

20 Shunmugam M, Azuara-Blanco A. The quality of reporting of diagnostic accuracy studies in glaucoma using the Heidelberg retina tomograph. *Inves Ophthalmol Vis Sci* 2006;47:2317-23.

21 Siddiqui MAR, Azuara-Blanco A, Burr J. The quality of reporting of diagnostic accuracy studies published in ophthalmic journals. *Br J Ophthalmol* 2005;89:261-5.

22 Rama KR, Poovali S, Apsingi S. Quality of reporting of orthopaedic diagnostic accuracy studies is suboptimal. *Clin Orthopaed Relat Res* 2006;447:237-46.

23 Smidt N, Rutjes AWS, Van Der Windt DA, Ostelo RWJG, Bossuyt PM, Reitsma JB, et al. Reproducibility of the STARD checklist: an instrument to assess the quality of reporting of diagnostic accuracy studies. *BMC Med Res Methodol* 2006;6:12.

24 Zafar A, Khan GI, Siddiqui MAR. The quality of reporting of diagnostic accuracy studies in diabetic retinopathy screening: a systematic review. *Clin Exp Ophthalmol* 2008;36:537-42.

25 Whiting P, Rutjes AWS, Reitsma JB, Bossuyt PMM, Kleijnen J. The development of QUADAS: a tool for the quality assessment of studies of diagnostic accuracy included in systematic reviews. *BMC Med Res Methodol* 2003;3:25.

26 Whiting PF, Bossuyt PMM, Sterne JAC, Deeks JJ, Reitsma H, Leeflang M, et al. Updating QUADAS: evidence to inform the development of QUADAS-2. Secondary updating. 2011. www.bris.ac.uk/quadas/resources/quadas2reportv4.pdf.

27 Simel DL, Feussner JR, DeLong ER, Matchar DB. Intermediate, indeterminate, and uninterpretable diagnostic test results. *Med Decis Making* 1987;7:107-14.

28 Kamath BM, Piccoli DA, Magee JC, Sokol RJ. Pancreatic insufficiency is not a prevalent problem in Alagille syndrome. *J Pediatr Gastroenterol Nutr* 2012;55:612-4.

29 Glaser JE, Chamarthy M, Haramati LB, Esses D, Freeman LM. Successful and safe implementation of a trinary interpretation and reporting strategy for V/Q lung scintigraphy. *J Nucl Med* 2011;52:1508-12.

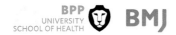

30 Ayad RF, Grayburn PA, Ko JM, Filardo G, Roberts WC. Accuracy of two-dimensional echocardiography in determining aortic valve structure in patients >50 years of age having aortic valve replacement for aortic stenosis. *Am J Cardiol* 2011;108:1589-99.

31 Delmas MC, Larsen C, van Benthem B, Hamers FF, Bergeron C, Poveda JD, et al. Cervical squamous intraepithelial lesions in HIV-infected women: prevalence, incidence and regression. *Aids* 2000;14:1775-84.

32 Begg CB,Greenes RA, Iglewicz B. The influence of uninterpretability on the assessment of diagnostic tests. *J Chronic Dis* 1986;39:575-84.

33 Coste J, Jourdain P, Pouchot J. A gray zone assigned to inconclusive results of quantitative diagnostic tests: application to the use of brain natriuretic peptide for diagnosis of heart failure in acute dyspneic patients. *Clin Chem* 2006;52:2229-35.

34 Santuz P, Soffiati M, Dorizzi RM, Benedetti M, Zaglia F, Biban P. Procalcitonin for the diagnosis of early-onset neonatal sepsis: a multilevel probabilistic approach. *Clin Biochem* 2008;41:1150-5.

35 Spencer JA. Indeterminate lesions in cancer imaging. *Clin Radiol* 2008;63:843-52.

36 Baloch ZW, Fleisher S, LiVolsi VA, Gupta PK. Diagnosis of "follicular neoplasm": a gray zone in thyroid fine-needle aspiration cytology. *Diagn Cytopathol* 2002;26:41-4.

37 Midthun K, Garrison L, Clements ML, Farzadegan H, Fernie B, Quinn T. Frequency of indeterminate western blot tests in healthy adults at low risk for human immunodeficiency virus infection. The NIAID AIDS Vaccine Clinical Trails Network. *J Infect Dis* 1990;162:1379-82.

38 Furukawa TA, Andrews G, Goldberg DP. Stratum-specific likelihood ratios of the general health questionnaire in the community: help-seeking and physical co-morbidity affect the test characteristics. *Psychol Med* 2002;32:743-8.

39 Straus SE RW, Glasziou P, Haynes BR. Evidence-based medicine: how to practice and teach EBM. Elsevier/Churchill Livingstone, 2005.

40 Blick CGT, Nazir SA, Mallett S, Turney BW, Onwu NN, Roberts ISD, et al. Evaluation of diagnostic strategies for bladder cancer using computed tomography (CT) urography, flexible cystoscopy and voided urine cytology: results for 778 patients from a hospital haematuria clinic. *BJU Int* 2012;110:84-94.

41 Poynard T, Chaput JC, Etienne JP. Relations between effectiveness of a diagnostic test, prevalence of the disease, and percentages of uninterpretable results. An example in the diagnosis of jaundice. *Med Decis Making* 1982;2:285-97.

42 Schuetz GM, Schlattmann P, Dewey M. Use of 3   2 tables with an intention to diagnose approach to assess clinical performance of diagnostic tests: meta-analytical evaluation of coronary CT angiography studies. *BMJ* 2012;345:e6717.

43 Subhas N, Sakamoto FA, Mariscalco MW, Polster JM, Obuchowski NA, Jones MH. Accuracy of MRI in the diagnosis of meniscal tears in older patients. *AJR Am J Roentgenol* 2012;198:575-80.

44 Rifkin RD. Maximum Shannon information content of diagnostic medical testing. Including application to multiple non-independent tests. *Med Decis Making* 1985;5:179-90.

45 Altman DG. The cost of dichotomising continuous variables. *BMJ* 2006;332:1080.

46 Knottnerus JA. The evidence base of clinical diagnosis. BMJ Publishing, 2002.

47 Sonis J. How to use and interpret interval likelihood ratios. *Fam Med J* 1999;31:432-7.

48 Peirce JC, Cornell RG. Integrating stratum-specific likelihood ratios with the analysis of ROC curves. *Med Decis Making* 1993;13:141-51.

49 Bowden SC, Loring DW. The diagnostic utility of multiple-level likelihood ratios. *J Int Neuropsychol Soc* 2009;15:769-76.

50 Furukawa TA, Goldberg DP, Rabe-Hesketh S, Ustun TB. Stratum-specific likelihood ratios of two versions of the General Health Questionnaire. *Psychol Med* 2001;31:519-29.

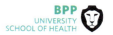

Making inferences on treatment effects from real world data: propensity scores, confounding by indication, and other perils for the unwary in observational research

Nick Freemantle, professor of clinical epidemiology and biostatistics[1][2],
Louise Marston, senior research statistician[1][2], Kate Walters, senior clinical lecturer in primary care and epidemiology[1], John Wood, principal research statistician[1][2],
Matthew R Reynolds, director, economics and quality of life research[3][4],
Irene Petersen, reader in epidemiology and statistics[1][2]

Department of Primary Care and Population Health, UCL Medical School (Royal Free Campus), London NW3 2PF, UK

MENT Clinical Trials Unit, UCL Medical School

Lahey Clinic Medical Center, Burlington, MA, USA

Harvard Clinical Research Institute, Boston, MA, USA

Correspondence to: nicholas. freemantle@ucl.ac.uk

Cite this as: BMJ 2013;347:f6409

doi: 10.1136/bmj.f6409

http://www.bmj.com/content/347/
bmj.f6409

For well rehearsed reasons, randomised trials are established as the mainstay of the evaluation of healthcare interventions. Indeed, as far back as 1935 Ronald Fisher commented that, "the simple act of randomisation assures the internal validity of the test for significance,"[1] before going on to lambast Charles Darwin for making strong conclusions from observational data. An irascible eugenicist and misogynist, Fisher was a brilliant but flawed genius; but we ignore his guidance on avoiding bias at our peril.

Though Fisher's aphorism remains true today, it addresses only part of the challenge. Decision makers could be equally interested in the external validity of a research finding, often asking for information about the effectiveness of treatments in the real world. Randomised trials, particularly those undertaken to support an application for marketing authorisation of a new medical product, may include by design only a stylised subset of patients with the particular condition: patients who are adherent and somewhat positively disposed to at least one of the treatment options (as identified by their agreement to be randomised); patients who are relatively lacking in comorbidities (to reduce the risk of serious adverse events that might confound the assessment of safety); and patients who are unrepresentatively young and often predominantly male (as investigators tend to be clinical specialists who draw from their local patient population, rather than generalists specialising in the complex problems of older people). Furthermore, participants are usually low risk because treatment is compared with a placebo (since the regulatory bodies require only proof that a product works not information on how it compares with existing treatments). Randomised trials are also expensive, with little change from $50m (£31m; €35m) for a landmark regulatory study, and they have a long lead time from inception to completion. This means that current patients with serious conditions may not benefit from the results even if the trials are conducted.

In attempts to address some of these limitations (trials conducted in the wrong or unrepresentative populations, or not done at all) researchers may turn to observational methods and the rich array of observational data to fill in some of the gaps.[2] In this paper we describe, through a series of examples, some of the potential advantages and perils of observational studies and suggest some strategies to negotiate the challenges safely.

ABSTRACT

Propensity score based methods are used increasingly to evaluate the effectiveness of treatments when evidence from randomised trials is not available. However, users need to be aware of their strengths and limitations

Propensity score analyses

Propensity scores were described by Rosenbaum and Rubin in 1983[3] as a deft means of accounting for known confounders or biases in estimation. They have developed a central place in observational research, being used in many settings, including those that do not lend themselves to randomised trials.[4] Smeeth et al used propensity score based analyses to address confounding in the comparison of people treated and not treated with statins.[5] Taking data from the Health Improvement Network (THIN), a data set based on general practice records, they fitted a statistical model to estimate the individual likelihood that patients would be prescribed a statin, using a list of 39 potential explanatory variables unaffected by exposure to statins, including demographic and medical history, prescribed drugs, social deprivation, and consultation behaviour. This provided a propensity score for each patient (that is, the model's prediction of the likelihood of receiving a statin). They used these scores to adjust for confounding when estimating the differences in outcome between patients receiving and not receiving statins but with a similar propensity for receiving statins. We can have some confidence that the adjustment using propensity scores was successful because their results were closely in line with those for vascular outcomes in randomised trials, lending support to the notion that other non-vascular outcomes (the focus of their research) may also reasonably be compared.

Propensity scores can be used for adjustment in statistical models or to create matched groups by selecting treatment and control patients with similar propensity scores. In both applications, propensity scores are used to account for known confounders and their use may lead to quite different results from those gleaned from unadjusted comparisons. Indeed, propensity score models can be considered a special case of multivariable adjustment. Propensity matched analyses are particularly attractive as they include in the analyses only participants who have a similar propensity score and thus baseline characteristics.

Matched propensity score evaluations also make it straightforward to compare the characteristics of treated and untreated groups and promote analysis strategies analogous to those used for randomised trials, although difficulties in achieving adequate matches may lead to small sample sizes and reduce external validity.

When things go awry

Although potentially helpful, the use of propensity scores does not assure the internal validity of the significance test, and decision makers need to be wary of making inferences from their results. This can be illustrated by the case of spironolactone, an aldosterone inhibitor that in the Randomized Aldactone Evaluation Study (RALES) reduced mortality in patients with severe heart failure (hazard ratio 0.70, 95% confidence interval 0.60 to 0.82, P<0.001).[6] The result was independently confirmed in two other trials.[7][8] Using a propensity score matching approach, we attempted to replicate the RALES trial[6] using data from the Health Improvement Network, with the ultimate objective of bridging from the trial population to a real world population of people with heart failure.[9] We included only patients who had recently been treated with high dose loop diuretics (.80 mg furosemide a day or equivalent), which indicates congestion, and excluded patients on the palliative care register, those with renal dysfunction, and those with recent cancer or unstable angina, liver failure, or a heart transplant. We used a large number of indicators of patient demography, comorbidities, and drug treatments to develop a propensity score. This was used to make two tightly matched groups of patients (n=4412) treated and not treated with spironolactone. We also did many supportive analyses, essentially taking a series of different defensible approaches to creating the propensity scores in order to explore consistency, adding further potential risk factors such as recent acute medical hospital admission and increasing the required precision by which matches were acceptable.

Survival in the spironolactone treated groups in RALES[6] and in our propensity matched study was remarkably similar, with just over 80% survival in both cohorts at one year. However, when we compared the tightly matched propensity score groups, rather than reducing mortality, spironolactone seemed to be associated with a substantial increase in the risk of death (figure). So must we conclude that spironolactone is dangerous in heart failure and should not be used, favouring the findings of the propensity matched analyses over those of the randomised clinical trials? Such strong conclusions have been drawn for other drugs on the basis of evidence of similar quality.[10][11] But we contend that such a conclusion would be quite unsafe. Below we explore some of the reasons why propensity score analyses may give incorrect answers.

Unknown bias

Randomisation, when properly conducted, avoi[ds] bias by distributing both known and unknown patie[nt] characteristics between the experimental conditions [on] the basis of the play of chance. This provides a good ba[sis] for comparison between the groups. It also underpins [our] statistical analyses because there are just two poten[tial] (orthogonal) explanations for any difference observ[ed] between the experimental groups: that the differences a[re] due either to the randomised treatment or to the play [of] chance. If it is implausible that chance is responsible [for] the observed difference because the P value is very small [or] the confidence intervals are a long way from the point of [no] difference, it must be due to the effects of treatment. It [is,] as Fisher recognised, a neat trick.

Propensity score based analyses, by contrast, accou[nt] only for known and observed patient characteristics. [We] hope that by balancing these known confounders we m[ay] derive an unbiased estimate of the effects of treatme[nt.] As Rosenbaum and Rubin pointed out in 1983,[3] this noti[on] requires the assumption that treatment assignment (in o[ur] case spironolactone or no spironolactone) is "otherwi[se] ignorable"—that is, that no additional unknown process[es] related to patient severity are associated with determini[ng] who will or will not receive treatment. Of course biases c[an] be found in randomised trials and propensity score analyse[s,] and both have the potential to be conducted poorly. F[or] example, attribution bias in non-blinded trials, loss [to] follow-up, or failure to follow the intention to treat princip[le] will all lead to biased results from randomised trials. [In] randomised trials and observational studies clinicians m[ay] introduce treatments considered in the best interest of t[he] patient but which could undermine the intended compariso[n.] For example, in the spironolactone study investigators m[ay] have introduced alternative treatments for heart failu[re] that were not adequately recorded (although we found [no] evidence of this). In randomised trials the investigators m[ay] (correctly) introduce treatments that undermine the validi[ty] of the trial comparison, while acting in the best interes[ts] of the patient. Both trials and propensity score analys[es] must be conducted to high methodological standard[s,] although ensuring this for propensity score analyses, whi[ch] are intrinsically more complex, can be harder.

The design of a study can sometimes make the decisi[on] to treat a patient "otherwise ignorable"—for example, in t[he] use of the propensity score to identify appropriate subjec[ts] to compare rhythm and rate control in an observation[al] study based on the AFFIRM trial.[12][13] In the AFFIRM tr[ial] participants were randomised to rhythm control drugs [or] rate control drugs, but the actual drug prescribed in th[at] class was determined by the investigator physician; t[he] AFFIRM investigators were comparing treatment strategi[es] (rate versus rhythm control) rather than individual drug[s.] However, Saksena and colleagues sought to use the[ir] data to make valid comparisons between particul[ar] antiarrhythmic drugs and the rate control strateg[y.] Although the doctor chose the antiarrhythmic—and so t[he] choice may carry information about severity—the decisi[on] not to use an antiarrhythmic drug is ignorable by desig[n] (because it was allocated on the play of chance). So simil[ar] comparator subjects should exist in the rate control grou[p] for each antiarrhythmic drug chosen, and propensity sco[re] matching should provide an excellent basis for identifyi[ng] control subjects. In a truly observational setting there [...]

	No of events	No of participants	Hazard ratio (95% CI)	P value	Hazard ratio (95% CI)
RALES 1999	670	1663		<0.001	0.70 (0.60 to 0.82)
Overall propensity score matched analysis	1285	4412		<0.001	1.32 (1.18 to 1.47)
Propensity score quartile >75% to 100%	369	1103		0.085	1.20 (0.98 to 1.47)
Propensity score quartile >50% to ≤75%	388	1103		0.91	0.99 (0.81 to 1.21)
Propensity score quartile >25% to ≤50%	298	1103		0.001	1.46 (1.16 to 1.83)
Propensity score quartile ≤25%	230	1103		<0.001	2.01 (1.54 to 2.63)

0.5 1 2 5

Fig Effect of spironolactone on mortality by all cause in RALES and propensity score analysis. Results for propensity analysis given overall and by quartile

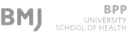

the potential risk that the choice of treatment is driven by patient characteristics, resulting in few if any control subjects being available, which reduces estimation precision and external validity.

Confounding by indication

Confounding by indication is the situation where allocation to treatment is not otherwise ignorable but instead subject to some latent (unrecognised or unmeasured) process associated with those who are treated—for example, when skilled clinicians use their expert judgment to decide whether to treat a patient and this judgment includes criteria describing the severity of the condition or the frailty of the patient not included in the propensity score or, more likely, not even formally measured. The challenge of a latent function such as confounding by indication is that it (by definition) cannot be measured directly but only tangentially through its effects, if it is recognised at all.

One obvious way to assess the performance of a propensity score is to examine its performance for homogeneity at different points on the propensity score scale.[14] In the figure we describe the effect of randomisation to spironolactone rather than placebo in the RALES trial,[6] then provide estimates derived from our propensity score matched model and for the four quartiles of the propensity scores used to generate the matched comparison. The hazard ratio for the overall propensity score analysis differs from that in the RALES trial by 6.4 standard errors (P<0.001), but there is also substantial variation between different values on the propensity score scale (test for interaction between the propensity score and spironolactone P=0.003).

Although the matched comparisons performed poorly for all values of the propensity scores, they were particularly misleading for participants who scored below the median likelihood of receiving spironolactone. One explanation for the spironolactone effects across the range of the scale, and in particular in the apparently low propensity subjects, is that the prescriber making the clinical decision to treat used additional important information on severity of heart failure that the propensity score did not capture, and so the match was made with inappropriately low risk individuals. In other words, the decision to prescribe was not otherwise ignorable.

When is it helpful to use a propensity score analysis?

Had the evidence for spironolactone from the RALES trial been less convincing we may have been tempted to conclude that spironolactone was indeed associated with substantial harm, and if that finding had been listened to, patients may have died who otherwise would have lived longer. There are certainly cases where patient harm seems likely because of the interpretation of propensity score analyses that are open to the risk of confounding by indication.[10] [11] [15]

The salutary example of our propensity matched analysis comparing patients who were treated with spironolactone and those who were not in patients with moderate to severe heart failure illustrates the perils for the unwary but also helps us to consider some rather limited strategies to identify or circumnavigate the problems.

Firstly, as confounding by indication is not directly measurable, this offers challenges to the analyst. Propensity score analysis will not lead to biased estimates of treatment effect if it is used in situations where the treatment decision is otherwise ignorable. For example, the analysis of the effects of statins by Smeeth et al[5] examined a treatment that tends to be used algorithmically based on estimated long term risk of major morbidity or mortality, rather than

in a response to observed patient morbidity, and so the treatment decision may be considered more likely to be otherwise ignorable.

Secondly, a useful precaution against unsafe inference from an observational study is to start with the replication of a known treatment effect and bridge from there to consider further, hitherto unanswered, questions. This was the approach taken in the analysis by Smeeth et al, who first replicated the vascular findings of the randomised trials before bridging to examine other outcomes of importance.[5] It was also our aim in the spironolactone analyses, where our intention was to bridge from a replication of the RALES trial to examine treatment effects in a broader group of patients, (women, those who are older, those with comorbidities and other different characteristics).

Thirdly, Rosenbaum and Rubin identified the potential importance of stratified analyses using propensity scores.[14] Our example shows both the usefulness of the test for interaction between propensity score and treatment effect and of describing the outcome of treatment across the range of propensity score values. If the propensity score analysis has worked as hoped we would expect to see a similar effect of 'treatment' across the range of propensity score values. If there are different effects for different propensity score values this should ring alarm bells, making it is a useful diagnostic.

Fourthly, and fundamentally, it is possible to identify important questions prospectively and conduct additional relevant randomised trials earlier, avoiding the need to rely on weaker methods. When clinicians need unbiased estimates of treatment effects among older people, women, or those with comorbidities, we should require answers to these questions from industry and publicly funded randomised trials.

Contributors: NF had the original idea for the paper, did the original statistical analyses described in the article, and wrote the first draft. JW aided in design. All authors revised the manuscript and approved the final version.

Competing interests: We have read and understood the BMJ policy on declaration of interests and have no relevant interests to declare.

Provenance and peer review: Not commissioned; externally peer reviewed.

1   Fisher RA. The design of experiments. 8th ed. Oliver and Boyd, 1966:21.
2   Avorn J. In defense of pharmacoepidemiology—embracing the yin and yang of drug research. N Engl J Med 2007;357:2219-21.
3   Rosenbaum PR, Rubin DB. The central role of the propensity score in observational studies for causal effects. Biometrika 1983;70:41-55.
4   Williamson E, Morley R, Lucas A, Carpenter J. Propensity scores: from naive enthusiasm to intuitive understanding. Stat Methods Med Res 2012;21:273-93.
5   Smeeth L, Douglas I, Hall AJ, Hubbard R, Evans S. Effect of statins on a wide range of health outcomes: a cohort study validated by comparison with randomized trials. Br J Clin Pharmacol 2008;67:99-109.
6   Pitt B, Annad FZ, Remme WJ, Cody R, Castaigne A, Perez A, et al. The effect of spironolactone on morbidity and mortality in patients with severe heart failure. N Engl J Med 1999;341:709-17.
7   Pitt B, Remme W, Zannad F, Neaton J, Martinez F, Roniker B, et al. Eplerenone, a selective aldosterone blocker, in patients with left ventricular dysfunction after myocardial infarction. N Engl J Med 2003;348:1309-21.
8   Zannad F, McMurray JJV, Krum H, van Veldhuisen DJ, Swedberg K, Shi H, et al. Eplerenone in patients with systolic heart failure and mild symptoms. N Engl J Med 2011;364:11-21.
9   Trends in the characteristics, treatment and prognosis of people with symptomatic heart failure and the use of aldosterone antagonists: analysis plan. www.ucl.ac.uk/priment/documents/Heart-Failure-Analysis-Plan.
10   Mangano DT, Tudor JC, Dietzel C. The risk associated with aprotinin in cardiac surgery. N Engl J Med 2006;354:353-65.
11   Mangano DT, Miao Y, Vuylsteke A, Tudor JC, Juneja R, Filipescu D, et al. Mortality associated with aprotinin during 5 years following coronary artery bypass graft surgery. JAMA 2007;297:471-9.
12   A comparison of rate control and rhythm control in patients with atrial fibrillation. N Engl J Med 2002;347:1825-33.

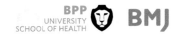

13   Saksena S, Slee A, Waldo AL, Freemantle N, Reynolds M, Rosenberg
     Y, et al. Cardiovascular outcomes in the AFFIRM trial: an assessment
     of individual antiarrhythmic drug therapies compared to rate
     control using propensity score matched analyses. *J Am Clin Cardiol*
     2011;19:1975-85.

14   Rosenbaum PR, Rubin DB. Reducing bias in observational studies
     using subclassification on the propensity score. *J Am Stat Assoc*
     1984;79:516-24.

15   Howell NJ, Senanayake EL, Freemantle N, Pagano D. Putting the
     record straight: aprotinin is safe and effective. Results from a mixed
     treatment meta-analysis of trials of aprotinin including the BART
     study. *J Thor Cardiovasc Surg* 2013;145:234-40.

More titles in
The BMJ Series

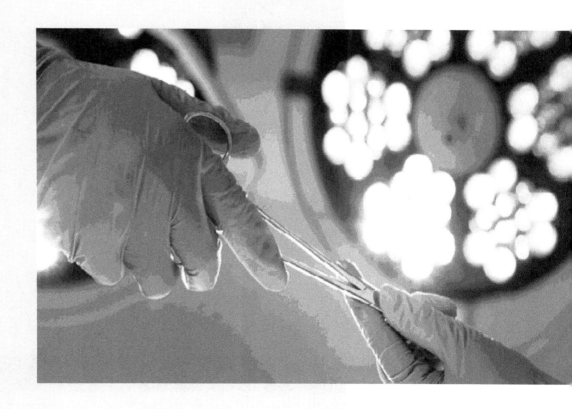

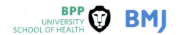
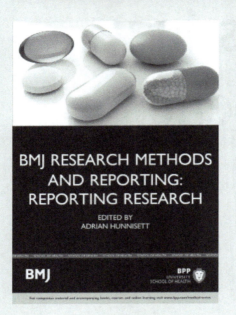
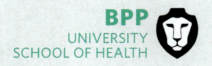

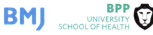

More titles in The BMJ Research Methods and Reporting Series

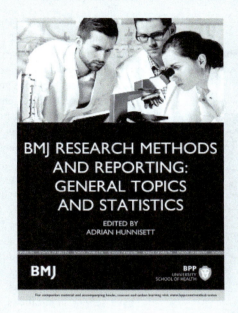

This book is the second of two volumes drawing together a collection of articles previously published in the BMJ covering contemporary issues in research. In this volume, the articles give key messages about how the 'nuts and bolts' of doing research, particularly with reference to how research findings should be reported. Each article also provides linked information and explicit evidence to support the statements made. The topics covered take a look at guidelines such as CONSORT, SPIRIT, GPP2, PRISMA and the IDEAL framework for surgical innovation. It also gives some guidance on economic evaluations, policy and service interventions and publication guidelines, as well as providing useful tips on preparing data for publication. Each article is written by an expert in the field and the volume brings together a masterclass in research reporting.

£29.99

May 2016

Paperback

978-1-472747-61-7

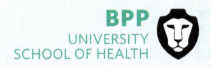

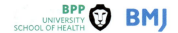
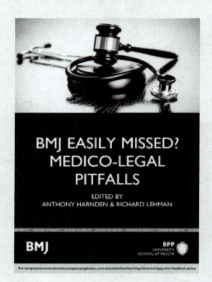
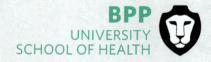

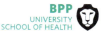
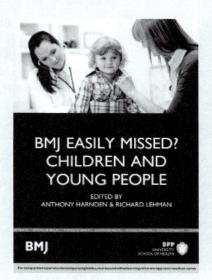
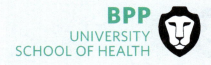

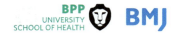

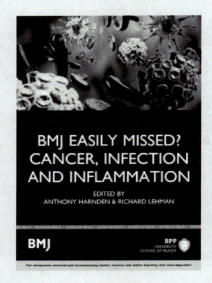

£29.99
January 2016
Paperback
978-1-472738-96-7

The risk of litigation against clinicians is increasing significantly. Those working in primary care, and whom are often dealing with uncertainty, are at particular risk. This book groups together a series of useful articles on diagnoses that may be easily missed at first presentation in primary care, and which may give rise to clinical negligence claims. The spectrum of conditions which are commonly encountered in claims such as pulmonary embolism, acute leg ischaemia, ectopic pregnancy, inflammatory bowel disease, appendicitis and achilles tendon rupture. All articles describe data to support the assertion that the conditions are often overlooked in primary care and that failure to recognise the diagnosis may have serious implications for the patient.

This book provides the reader with:

- Diagnoses that may be encountered in clinical negligence claims
- Evidence that the diagnoses are easily missed in primary care
- Succinct articles with specific learning points and take home messages
- Essential reading to reduce risk of future litigation

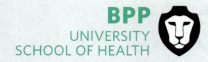

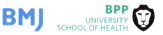
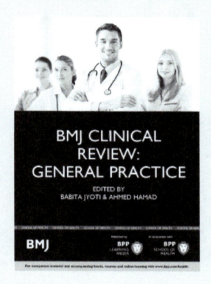
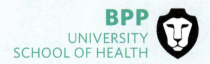

More titles from BPP School of Health

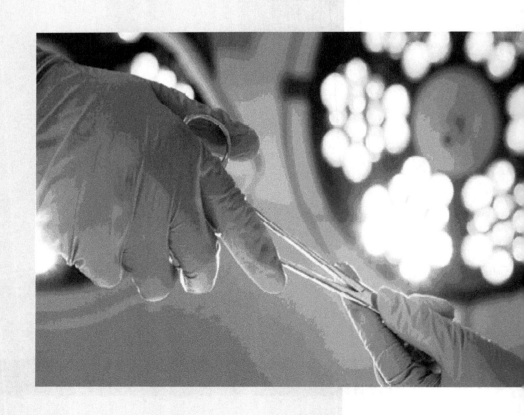

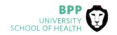

More titles in The Progressing your Medical Career Series

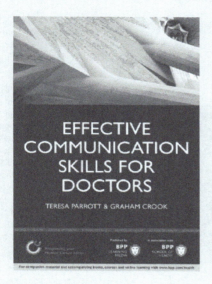

£19.99
September 2011
Paperback
978-1-445379-56-2

Would you like to know how to improve your communication skills? Are you looking for a clearly written book which explores all aspects of effective medical communication?

There is an urgent need to improve doctors' communication skills. Research has shown that poor communication can contribute to patient dissatisfaction, lack of compliance and increased medico-legal problems. Improved communication skills will impact positively on all of these areas.

The last fifteen years have seen unprecedented changes in medicine and the role of doctors. Effective communication skills are vital to these new roles. But communication is not just related to personality. Skills can be learned which can make your communication more effective, and help you to improve your relationships with patients, their families and fellow doctors.

This book shows how to learn those skills and outlines why we all need to communicate more effectively. Healthcare is increasingly a partnership. Change is happening at all levels, from government directives to patient expectations. Communication is a bridge between the wisdom of the past and the vision of the future.

Readers of this book can also gain free access to an online module which upon successful completion can download a certificate for their portfolio of learning/ Revalidation/ CPD records.

This easy-to-read guide will help medical students and doctors at all stages of their careers improve their communication within a hospital environment.

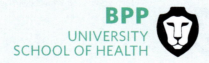

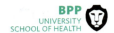

More titles in The Progressing your Medical Career Series

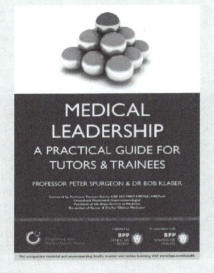

£19.99

November 2011

Paperback

978-1-445379-57-9

Are you a doctor or medical student who wishes to acquire and develop your leadership and management skills? Do you recognise the role and influence of strong leadership and management in modern medicine?

Clinical leadership is something in which all doctors should have an important role in terms of driving forward high quality care for their patients. In this up-to-date guide Peter Spurgeon and Robert Klaber take you through the latest leadership and management thinking, and how this links in with the Medical Leadership Competency Framework. As well as influencing undergraduate curricula and some of the concepts underpinning revalidation, this framework forms the basis of the leadership component of the curricula for all medical specialties, so a practical knowledge of it is essential for all doctors in training.

Using case studies and practical exercises to provide a strong work-based emphasis, this practical guide will enable you to build on your existing experiences to develop your leadership and management skills, and to develop strategies and approaches to improving care for your patients.

This book addresses:

- Why strong leadership and management are crucial to delivering high quality care
- The theory and evidence behind the Medical Leadership Competency Framework
- The practical aspects of leadership learning in a wide range of clinical environments (eg handover, EM, ward etc)
- How Consultants and trainers can best facilitate leadership learning for their trainees and students within the clinical work-place

Whether you are a medical student just starting out on your career, or an established doctor wishing to develop yourself as a clinical leader, this practical, easy-to-use guide will give you the techniques and knowledge you require to excel.

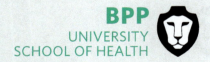

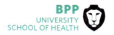

More Titles in The Progressing Your Medical Career Series

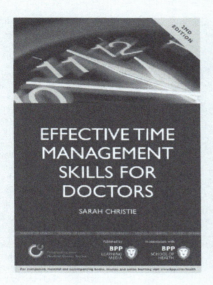

£19.99

February 2012

Paperback

978-1-445390-15-4

Do you find it difficult to achieve a work-life balance? Would you like to know how you can become more effective with the time you have?

With the introduction of the European Working Time Directive, which will severely limit the hours in the working week, it is more important than ever that doctors improve their personal effectiveness and time management skills. This interactive book will enable you to focus on what activities are needlessly taking up your time and what steps you can take to manage your time better.

By taking the time to read through, complete the exercises and follow the advice contained within this book you will begin to:

- Understand where your time is being needlessly wasted

- Discover how to be more assertive and learn how to say 'No'

- Set yourself priorities and stick to them

- Learn how to complete tasks more efficiently

- Plan better so you can spend more time doing the things you enjoy

In recent years, with the introduction of the NHS Plan and Lord Darzi's commitment to improve the quality of healthcare provision, there is a need for doctors to become more effective within their working environment. This book will offer you the chance to regain some clarity on how you actually spend your time and give you the impetus to ensure you achieve the tasks and goals which are important to you.

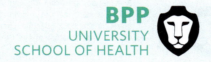

BPP
UNIVERSITY
SCHOOL OF HEALTH

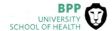

More titles in The Essential Clinical Handbook Series

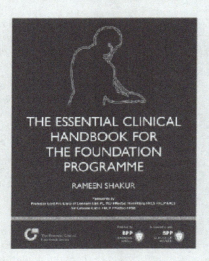

THE ESSENTIAL CLINICAL HANDBOOK FOR THE FOUNDATION PROGRAMME

RAMEEN SHAKUR

£24.99

October 2011

Paperback

978-1-445381-63-3

Unsure of what clinical competencies you must gain to successfully complete the Foundation Programme? Unclear on how to ensure your ePortfolio is complete to enable your progression to ST training?

This up-to-date clinical handbook is aimed at current foundation doctors and clinical medical students and provides a comprehensive companion to help you in the day-to-day management of patients on the ward. Together with this it is the first handbook to also outline clearly how to gain the core clinical competencies required for successful completion of the Foundation Programme. Written by doctors for doctors this comprehensive handbook explains how to successfully manage all of the common cases you will face during the Foundation Programme and:

- Introduces the Foundation Programme and what is expected of a new doctor especially with the introduction of Modernising Medical Careers

- Illustrates clearly the best way to manage, step-by-step, over 150 commonly encountered clinical diseases, including NICE guidelines to ensure a gold standard of clinical care is achieved

- Describes how to successfully gain the core clinical competencies within Medicine and Surgery including an extensive list of differentials and conditions explained

- Explores the various radiology images you will encounter and how to interpret them

- Tells you how to succeed in the assessment methods used including DOP's, Mini-CEX's and CBD's

- Has step by step diagrammatic guide to doing common clinical procedures competently and safely

- Outlines how to ensure your ePortfolio is maintained properly to ensure successful completion of the Foundation Programme

- Provides tips and advice on how to start preparing now to ensure you are fully prepared and have the competitive edge for your CMT/ST application

The introduction of the e-Portfolio as part of the Foundation Programme has paved the way for foundation doctors to take charge of their own learning and portfolio. Through following the expert guidance laid down in this handbook you will give yourself the best possible chance of progressing successfully through to CMT/ST training.

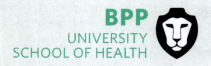

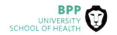

More titles in The Essential Clinical Handbook Series

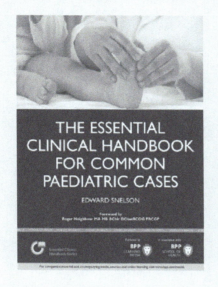

£24.99

September 2011

Paperback

978-1-445379-60-9

Not sure what to do when faced with a crying baby and demanding parent on the ward? Would you like a definitive guide on how to manage commonly encountered paediatric cases?

This clear and concise clinical handbook has been written to help healthcare professionals approach the initial assessment and management of paediatric cases commonly encountered by Junior Doctors, GPs, GP Specialty Trainee's and allied healthcare professionals. The children who make paediatrics so fun, can also make it more than a little daunting for even the most confident person. This insightful guide has been written based on the author's extensive experience within both a General Practice and hospital setting.

Intended as a practical guide to common paediatric problems it will increase confidence and satisfaction in managing these conditions. Each chapter provides a clear structure for investigating potential paediatric illnesses including clinical and non-clinical advice covering: background, how to assess, pitfalls to avoid, FAQs and what to tell parents. This helpful guide provides:

- A problem/symptom based approach to common paediatric conditions

- As essential guide for any doctor assessing children on the front line

- Provides easy-to-follow and step-by-step guidance on how to approach different paediatric conditions

- Useful both as a textbook and a quick reference guide when needed on the ward

This engaging and easy to use guide will provide you with the knowledge, skills and confidence required to effectively diagnose and manage commonly encountered paediatric cases both within a primary and secondary care setting.

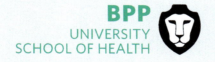

www.bpp.com/medical-series

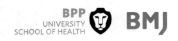